PALEO COOKBOOK FOR BEGINNERS

QUICK AND EASY RECIPES TO LOSE WEIGHT AND GET INTO SHAPE

FRANCESCA BONHEUR

APEX UNIVERSAL PTY LTD

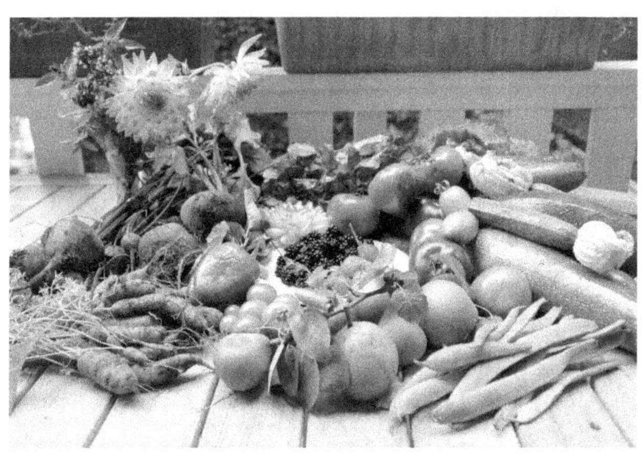

DEDICATION AND GRATITUDE

If this Paleo cookbook shall be dedicated to someone, it should be dedicated to each man and woman or even child who are trying to resist the strong authority of packaged foods. Throughout the entire process of writing this informative book, many people from the community have granted us from their precious time to help us come out with this content. We want to thank you for your active participation in this book either by sharing your personal point of view or by sharing this book with your friends.

CONTENTS

ABOUT THIS BOOK

When people tend to adopt a new living method and a new diet; they might be looking for the best way to help them feel better and live healthier; this is not an assumption, but rather a truth. Indeed, we can call Paleo diet the unique lifestyle choice par excellence that encourages the consumption of certain foods more than other types of food. And what characterizes this specific type of diet is that it is also based on eating food like our ancestors did; based on an evolutionary perspective. Some other people would adopt a new form of diet because of different personal reasons like remaining fit as long as they can. And one of the most important reasons for adopting a Paleo diet is that it increases autoimmunity and provides the body with a high load of protein, low carbohydrates and completely natural nutrients. The focus in this book, titled *"Lose Weight with Paleo Diet for Beginners"* will be mainly destined to guide you to the best diet you should adopt in order to benefit as much as possible from Paleo Diet. This book will also allow you not only to learn how to adopt a brand-new Paleo lifestyle in order to feel healthy, lose weight, and also increase the level of energy. With this Paleo cookbook for Beginners, you will have the healthiest life you have ever dreamt of. Besides, you will be able to reduce any diabetes problems you might be suffering from like heart diseases and cancer as well as modern ailments. This Paleo Cookbook for Beginners is a straightaway, guide that will make you succeed in embracing and living according to a new diet. In this book, you will also find a daily plan that will help you know what you should eat throughout the entire day, especially if you are a beginner. So, if you are new to Paleo diet and you can't wait to start, get ready to read the most informative Paleo guiding cookbook you can find. In addition to a brief history about the origins of Paleo Diets, you will find everything you need to know about the recommended ingredients you should use and the main ingredients you should exclude from your diet.

CHAPTER 1

INTRODUCTION

I WANT to thank you and congratulate you for downloading the book, titled *"Lose weight with Paleo Diet Cookbook for Beginners"*. Welcome to this Paleo Cookbook Diet; if you have chosen our book, then you have picked up the right book to help you adopt one of the most beneficial dietary programs you can find. And even if you are a beginner in adopting Paleo Diet and you don't know where to start from, then this book will lead your way in finding all the information you need to explain to you the major basics of Paleo Diet. You will also be able to understand what makes a type of food called a Paleo Food and what sets it apart from other types of food. You will learn that Paleo food comprises the healthiest food ingredients. And although we might not know what the main reason that encouraged you to adopt this specific dietary food habit is; we congratulate you because this is the best choice you have ever made. And no matter who suggested Paleo Diet for you, he or she has set you for the best dietary path you can choose in order to help you remain healthy and safe. If you also found this book hazardously and you don't have any idea what it is about; then rest assured because we will cover this topic in a detailed way. We encourage you to carefully read our book chapter by chapter so that you understand all the parts and the steps of a Paleo Dietary program. And whether you want to lose weight or eat healthy; you will learn how to improve each part of your body. You can also call this book, your Daily Plan of Paleo diet Cookbook; the book that will inspire you to enjoy each meal you have. Some people might think that they are wasting their money and time by adopting such a Paleo diet; but you will find that Paleo Recipes are very easy to make. And this book will show you what makes a Paleo diet very healthy and it will teach you how to avoid eating harmful food ingredients. And when we say Paleo diet, we are speaking about autoimmunity protocol; this protocol classifies ingredients into two sets; the first includes the food ingredients we should eat and the second includes the list of food ingredients we should remove from our daily meals. This "Paleo Diet Cookbook for Beginners" will lead your way in your journey to discover the Paleo Foods that you shall eat in order to improve your immunity system and to decrease any serious infection or risk of inflammation that can affect you. What is more surprising and pleasing about Paleo diet is that you won't need a long time to cook Paleo Recipes; and in addition to the delicious recipes you will read; you will learn many tips that can improve your health in a matter of a few days. We will try to explain to you how to get used to a new, economic and easy diet. Don't worry if you don't even know how to fry an egg or cook a simple meal because we will help you learn how to be a cook in a very short time. With a wide range of recipes and a variety of ingredients, we will offer you some of the most scrumptious dishes from chicken recipes to Beef Recipes to Vegan Recipes, Vegetarian Recipes, fish, seafood Recipes and more. If you have a health problem; then this book will be able to reverse any risk that may endanger your health and you will enjoy every meal. All the recipes you will find in this book are all made by a professional cook and created with extra care and love. So if you want to change your life for the better and to improve your life condition; this book is yours. You will still be able to enjoy your conventional delicious recipes that you thought you have to give up on. Consider this book, your own collection of nourishing and succulent recipes, that are completely seeds-free, grain-free, dairy-free and gluten free. We hope that you will like our book and if you are ready to take up the challenge, and then let us get started.

CHAPTER 2

WHAT IS PALEO DIET?

HEALTH BENEFITS OF WHOLE FOODS AND HEALTH ISSUES OF WITH PACKAGED FOOD AND OBESITY IN AMERICA

THE TERM PALEO is derived from the word Palaeolithic and it was later developed into what we call today a Paleo Diet. Some researchers believe that the Paleo diet originates from Greek while other scientists believe that Paleo diet was known as the Stone Age, diet or the diet of Cavemen; and it literally means the diet that our ancestors adopted thousands of years ago. Paleo diet is based on a preset diet that our ancestors had followed even without knowing around 2 and half million of years ago. This specific stone aged diet is based on including only natural types of food and on excluding any food ingredients that are chemically processed. And in order to better understand the meaning of a Paleo Diet, we should have a glance at the history of Paleo diet and how it evolved in our contemporary time; especially that Paleo diet has become one of the most important dietary trends nowadays.

The idea of the Paleo diet originates from the natural food that are provided to us directly from the nature just like the ancestors lived more than 10 thousand years ago. Our ancestors ate no beans, no cereals, no potatoes; no dairy products or milk and no sugar at all.

Many scientists were interested in Paleo Diets and studied it very closely. Indeed, the study of the diets of our ancestors is called nutritional anthropology science. Some other scientists refer the Paleo diet to the Palaeolithic era during the history of humanity.

What also drew the scientists' attention to Paleo diet was that primitive people, who ate natural food, didn't suffer modern diseases like obesity, cancer and diabetes. So there is no doubt that the Paleo Diet is one of the most favourite forms of diet for the majority of the people. Yet, what are the benefits of Paleo Diet? What do the Paleo People eat and what do they drink? Each of us can choose the diet that fits us; some of us adopt the Paleo diet for a diversity of reasons and based on our health condition. And one of the most important reasons that urge people to adopt Paleo Diet is the autoimmune disease. In fact, it is believed that the Paleo Diet is one of the most effective natural ways to cure autoimmunity. And when we say autoimmune disease, we are speaking about autoimmune protocol. The Autoimmune Protocol is a very specialised version that displays the Paleo diet and it relies on a strict daily food plan. Food within a Paleo diet is divided into two main categories based on its ingredients. The first category of ingredients promotes our heath condition and the second category causes certain serious inflammations that can result in a serious degradation of our health. Scientists call the harmful food ingredients inflammatory compounds and the only effective way that was proved by nutritionists to prevent many diseases and inflammations is choosing Paleo Diet amongst all the other forms of diets. There are many benefits associated with Paleo Diet and weight loss is one of the most valued benefits that people are seeking. A scientific study has shown that most of the people embrace specific diets because they want to lose weight. And you might have adopted certain diets, but maybe you haven't lost as much weight as you imagined or maybe you lost weight; then gained more in a short period of time. The Paleo Diet is different and it has many other benefits in addition to weight loss.

CHAPTER 3

BENEFITS OF THE PALEO DIET

EACH OF US has probably heard about the Paleo diet except that we might not know what it exactly means. The Paleo diet that is also called the Caveman diet is the only diet that is based on eating meat, fresh vegetables and sugar- free ingredients. The Paleo Diet is believed to be one of the healthiest diets because of the plethora of benefits it provides. A recent study has determined that a person adopting a Pale Diet starts experiencing an improvement in their health condition during the early days. So what are the major benefits of a Paleo diet?

1. **The Paleo diet reduces the level of glucose in the blood.**

The main characteristic of the Paleo Diet is that it is sugar-free and it helps you avoid the constant consumption of refined sugar. And if you avoid including sugar in your dietary habits, it becomes easy to avoid a probable increase in the level of glucose. The Paleo diet won't let you feel any fatigue; yet, if you suffer from a diabetic condition, you still need to consult your doctor to see if you can adopt this diet.

1. **With the Paleo Diet, say goodbye to hunger**

Unlike most of the diets that make you feel very hungry all the time; the Paleo Diet focuses on making you feel full all the time. The majority of the people like this characteristic of the Paleo Diet as it help you feel satiety easily with the high amount of proteins and healthy fats that it provides. So, if you choose the Paleo diet, you will make sure that you are eating the best ingredients that are packed with proteins from meat and vitamins from veggies.

1. **With the Paleo Diet, no need for calorie count**

Unlike any other diet, in which you should keep watching the smart points and counting the carbohydrates that you need to consume daily, a Paleo Diet is easy to adapt to. The daily plan of Paleo diet is very easy because you can simply eat like the first human beings on earth did, without any complicated additives and ingredients.

1. **Reduces bloating**

Paleo diet is known for providing loads of fibres and a very small amount of sodium, which helps the body getting rid of bloating. In addition to preventing bloating, Paleo diet helps improve the digestion mechanisms and it relieves any digestive issues.

1. **Paleo Diet relieves fatigue**

Paleo diet helps relieving the body from the feelings of fatigue, fogginess and disorientation. The Paleo meals are made of high count of proteins and help our body get the body from the fats.

1. **Paleo Diet prevents many diseases**

When you adopt a certain diet, you choose to eat healthier food that contains anti-inflammatory ingredients and antioxidants. Thereby, you ensure getting the Phytonutrients that are necessary in preventing the risk of serious illnesses like cancer and cardiac disease. Paleo diet is based more on eating natural food rather than junk food.

1. **Paleo Diet can help relieve stress and improve your sleep**

By stopping including the chemicals and the additives into the sources of your food; then you will feel naturally tired and you will sleep normally and naturally at night. Your brain will be releasing serotonin as a signal to sleep better. This improves your health and will organize your internal rhythm, the way our ancestors did.

- **NOTE**

If you have chosen to follow the Paleo diet; then you would want to discover more about this topic and to learn everything that might help you understand what a Paleo Diet consists of and how it affects your life. And you should keep in mind that eating according to a Paleo diet doesn't mean an immediate loss of weight; yet it remains a great way to start trying to lose extra weight.

CHAPTER 4

HEALTH ISSUES OF PACKAGED FOODS AND OBESITY IN AMERICA

TO UNDERSTAND BETTER the relationship between packaged food and the problem of obesity in America, we should at first, try to figure out what overweight means and whom we can call obese. In general, nutritionists and specialists classify any population into four main categories, the first focuses on the people who are underweight, the second focuses on people who have a perfect, healthy weight and the third deals with people who are overweight and the fourth deals with people who suffer from obesity. The method according to which we can categorize people according to their weight is by following the body mass index or what we can the measurement of fat within our bodies based on our weight and our height. To help you understand better this idea, below is a chart that displays to you the basic approximate numbers, based on weight and height.

Category	The range of weight	Height	Body Mass Index
Underweight category	About 124 pounds	5′ 9″	Underneath 18.4
Healthy weight	From 125 pounds to about 168 pounds	5′ 9″	18.4 to 24.8
Over weighted category	From 69 pounds to 202 pounds	5′ 9″	25.1 to 29.7
Obesity category	203 pounds or more	5′ 9″	31.1 or higher

The figures in this table are approximate, but they are very reasonable and help us understand better in which range we can set ourselves and to know the exact answers to what make some of us overweight. What is most frustrating about obesity in the United States of America is that more than 37% of the American adults suffer from obesity. And a recent American study has reported that most of the American population is classified as overweight. The high rate of overweight in the United States of America urged the U.S health centres to classify obesity as a disease in order to find a way to prevent and control the problem of overweight and obesity. And according to official resources, the medical costs of fighting obesity in the USA, hit the roof of more than 147$ in the summer of 2008. And as there was no efficient way to prevent obesity, researchers and nutritionists advised people to start adopting healthy diets and exercise to lose weight. And one of the most effective diets is Paleo Diet. Yet, many other researchers focused on studying the main reason that might be responsible for obesity. The results scientists and nutritionists have found were conflicting, but at last, all the studies led to one and only conclusion; too much packed and junk food with very little exercise.

Junk food and the huge quantity of packaged or canned food, candies and soft drinks are the main ingredients that are driving the American society towards obesity. The noticeable increase in the consumption of packaged food through the United Stated has urged nutritionists to study its disadvantages on our eating habits. Packaged food led to a notable increase in the intake of toxins within the body. And although packaged food has some positive effects; it has a lot of disadvantages on our health.

1. **High in glucose and sugar**

Many of the packaged foods are known for containing high amounts of sugar. Consuming sugar more than our body needs can cause a diversity of diseases that can risk our lives like heart diseases, cholesterol; tooth decay and especially, obesity.

1. **Packaged food is packed with Sodium**

Packaged foods contain a very high level of sodium and salt; and while it is true that the salt plays an important role in preserving our foods, it can also cause serious health conditions. In fact, the high sodium in packaged food causes the elevation of the blood pressure and it increases the loss of calcium.

1. **Packaged food is rich in Trans fats**

Packaged food is rich in Trans fat that helps give the body a longer life on our shelves; but at the same time, it causes a serious increase in the level of cholesterol. Trans fats also threaten our lives with the heart diseases it causes. People, who consume more packaged foods, are more likely to suffer a heart stroke because of the high level of saturated fats.

1. **Additives and packaged food**

Additives are usually used in order to improve the shelf life of packaged food and to make the taste better, but not all the additives are safe to be used and most of the used additives are not considered to be safe by the American Drug and Food administration. So in order to avoid consuming such dangerous elements, we should pay more attention and purchase healthier ingredients rather than packaged food rich in additives.

- **NOTE:**

Losing weight remains one of the most difficult tasks that we try to achieve and the best way is to follow a healthy and safe diet, and we can't find better than a Paleo Diet to achieve this. You may ask yourself the question; why would you choose the Paleo Diet and not any other type of diet and the answer is very simple; Paleo Diet guarantees a weight loss in a short period of time. But before starting with the Paleo diet recipes, we should at first, know the list of ingredients we should use and the list of ingredients we should avoid when we adopt a Paleo Diet.

CHAPTER 5

LIST OF FOOD THAT YOU SHOULD INCLUDE IN YOUR PALEO DIET

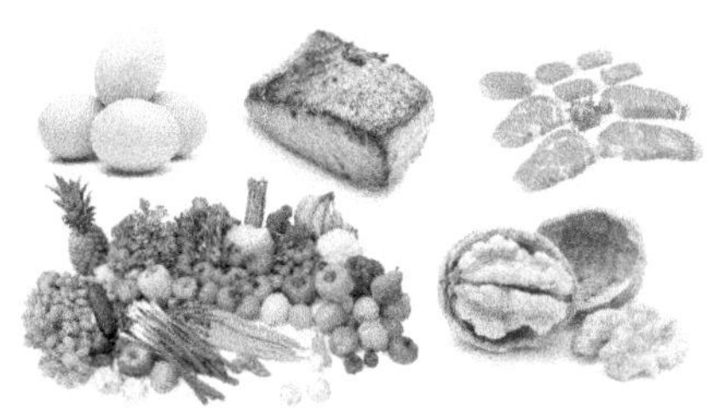

List of food that you should include in your Paleo Diet	List of food that you should exclude from your Paleo Diet
All vegetables; just make sure to avoid rice and corn wheat	Don't use Grains like quinoa
All fruits	Don't use legumes at all like peanuts and soy
Organ meats and the remaining types of meats	Don't use sugar
Using bone broth is advisable	Don't use any vegetable or oils of seeds
Seafood ingredients	Avoid using Additives and avoid all types of processed foods
Fermented foods	Don't use nuts
All healthy Fats	Don't use seeds like cocoa seeds, coffee and seed-based spices
Certain herbs	Avoid consuming nightshades like tomatoes, Aubergine, eggplants, potatoes, peppers and spices
Seeds	
Nuts	Avoid Alcohol
Healthy types of oil like walnut oil, avocado oil, coconut oil, flaxseed oil and macadamia oil	Don't use aspirin
	Avoid Stevia
Seafood, fish	Avoid using thickeners like guar gum and carrageenan; don't use algae too
Green leafy vegetables	
Root vegetables	

Learning the basic ingredients in Paleo Diet is not the only thing we should learn before adopting it. Indeed, a new diet is no exception and the hardest part is to set the first step into this new journey. The Paleo diet relies on new adjustments and on exercising at the same time.

So are you ready to learn how keep your Paleo diet simple and to stick to our plan? It is very simple; just follow our dietary plan based on a high level of protein intake; mainly on meat and fish with whole foods and a plenty of non-starchy vegetables. Although you have to give up on the delicious staples you used to eat, you are going to enjoy our healthy Paleo recipes. And if you chose the Paleo Diet to lose weight, just make sure to use only a few ingredients and avoid adding too many additives and flavours.

CHAPTER 6

PALEO RECIPES AND WEIGHT LOSS

THE PALEO DIET has proven to be the diet number one in achieving great results as far as weight loss is concerned. And according to a nutritional study, the Paleo diet has been ranked as the best diet out of about thirty one diets. The very good results of the Paleo Diet encourage us to question the main role it plays in weight loss. And although many nutritional experts believe that the Paleo Diet is hard to follow; others have proved that the Paleo Diet is the best diet that leads to weight loss based on the several tips below:

1. **Make sure to eat what you need, no more, no less**

Many followers of a Paleo Diet think that eating less food is the shortest way to lose weight; but this belief is not true. Excluding many types of food ingredients may deprive your body from necessary elements and substantial nutrients that provide the energy for the body. Thereby, a wrong approach of following the Paleo Diet may lead to certain deficiencies like iron deficiency and other illnesses Many Paleo believe that less food is always better when it comes to losing weight. Besides, decreasing the intake of the calories the body needs may result in lowering the metabolic rate, which can defined as the number of calories we burn. You should understand that a dieting program doesn't mean to starve ourselves to death. What sets the Paleo Diet special is that it focuses on managing hunger and start to consume fewer calories. And this is one of the most important reasons that urge people to adopt the Paleo Diet instead of following any other form of diet.

Many Paleo Diet followers have experienced the good effects of the Paleo Diet and they lost pounds while at the same time, they enjoyed the same delicious food varieties.

1. **With Paleo diet, there is no need to complicate your food ingredients**

Many nutritional studies have proven that eating food with simple ingredients can help you lose weight without making so much effort. If you want to keep your food simple with simple ingredients; follow a daily meal plan rich in proteins like fish or meat. Try to consume the vegetables that are not starchy. So how do you keep a Paleo diet simple? Stick to the basics of a healthy meal.

1. **Don't start a Paleo Diet by yourself.**

One of the worst ways in trying to adopt a certain diet is to lose weight by you. Following the Paleo Diet in the right way can help you succeed and change your lifestyle for the better. You can make our recipes and even share it with your friends. And if you don't have anyone to help you and support you with your diet; you can find many groups of people who are following Paleo diets and who can help you.

1. **Paleo diet changes not only your eating habits, your lifestyle**

Choosing to adopt a Paleo Diet is a program not only focuses on losing weight, but also on changing your lifestyle to the better. Indeed, adopting Paleo Diet helps you sleep better and decreases the hormones of stress. Paleo diet also teaches you to improve the feeling of responsibility and helps you learn ways to manage your mind techniques better. When you follow a Paleo diet, you will be able to enjoy your everyday life better than you used to before following a Paleo Diet.

1. **Don't sit too much and make sure to move throughout the day**

Staying too much in the same place while you are on a Paleo Diet may endanger your health, especially if you have to work into your office or drive for long hours. So, in order to make the best results from your Paleo Diet, avoid sitting for a long time; and start exercising according to a daily plan. Try to walk for about thirty minutes per day to improve the risk of any possible disease.

Days	BREAKFAT	LUNCH	SNACK	DINNER
Sunday	Scrambled eggs with vegetables and bacon	Salad with taco	Fruits	baked sea bass with capers and lemon, with steamed broccoli
Monday	Stir fried sausage	The leftover of taco salad	pb&j	Sweet potatoes and chicken with sautéed kale and shallots
Tuesday	Simple salad	Sweet potatoes and leftover chicken	Vegetables and deli meat	Broccoli and beef
Wednesday	Omelet	Leftover broccoli and beef	Trail mix	Pork chops with bread with asparagus; roasted
Thursday	Oatmeal and chicken sausage	The leftover of pork chops and the roasted asparagus	Jerky and trail mix	Cutlets of chicken with tomatoes and olives with spaghetti squash with toasted almonds
Friday	Avocado salsa with eggs	Leftovers of Cutlets of chicken with tomatoes and olives with spaghetti squash with toasted almonds	Fruit and jerky	Turkey with cilantro and burgers + Green, roasted beans
Saturday	About 4 bacon with zucchini fritters	Leftovers of graze	Leftovers of graze	Vegetable chili and chill

- **NOTE:**

Following the Paleo diet will, for sure, help you lose weight, but you should make sure to make a plan before starting it and to learn some of the best and easy Paleo recipes. And to achieve the best results, make sure not to come back home with your stomach filled with junk and packaged food. In addition to this book, we have also a wide range of books that we have written with extra care about different types of diets. So, if you are interested in our recipes, feel free to download it. And remember that a good weight loss diet program does not necessarily rely on the count of calories, but rather about how organized your daily meal plan is. So starving yourself is not the best alternative; you should rather focus on dealing with your essential metabolic issues.

CHAPTER 7

PALEO CHICKEN RECIPES

CHICKEN DRUMSTICKS WITH COCONUT MILK

- ***Cooking Time: 40 minutes***
- ***Preparation Time: 5 minutes***
- ***Servings: 4-5***

- **NOTE:**

HAVE you just started your new Paleo diet and you feel hungry? And even if you are not hungry, you are going to like the mouthwatering taste of the golden chicken drumsticks. If this is your first Paleo diet recipe, you are going to enjoy it.

INGREDIENTS:

- 9 Chicken drumsticks
- 2 Cups of almond flour
- ½ Cup of Dijon mustard;
- ½ Cup of full-fat coconut milk
- 1 Tablespoon of lemon juice
- 4 Minced garlic cloves
- ½ Tablespoons of fresh thyme

- 2 Tablespoons of fresh lemon zest
- ¼ Cup of olive oil
- 1 Pinch of sea salt
- 1 Pinch of freshly ground black pepper

Directions

1. Preheat your oven to about 400 degree Fahrenheit
2. In a large and deep bowl, combine altogether the lemon juice with the coconut milk, lemon juice and the mustard.
3. Add the mixture of the mustard to the chicken and toss very well until your ingredients are very well-coated.
4. In a separate bowl; combine the garlic with the thyme, the lemon zest, and the almond meal; then adjust the seasoning with the salt and the pepper to taste.
5. Dip each of the chicken pieces into the mixture of the almond; then put the drumsticks
6. Put the chicken drumsticks over a baking sheet; then bake the chicken into the oven for about 40 minutes
7. Set the chicken aside to rest for about 5 minutes, then serve and enjoy it!

Nutritional information

- Calories per serving – 139 calories
- Fat per serving – 7.18 grams
- Saturated Fats – 1.95 gram
- Total Carbs per serving –0 grams
- Protein per serving – 17.4 grams

CHICKEN CHUNKS WITH GREEN ONION

- ***Cooking Time: 10 minutes***
- ***Preparation Time: 4 minutes***
- ***Servings: 2-3***

- **NOTE:**

This Paleo chicken meal is delicious and sticky. It is the best chicken meal you can enjoy with the coconut aminos. You can share this recipe with your family and with your friends too. It is a perfect chicken meal to serve on special occasions.

INGREDIENTS:

- 1 Pound of boneless and skinless chicken breast, diced into small chunks
- 7 Dried red chilies
- 3 Sliced green onions
- ¼ Cup of coconut aminos;
- 1 Tablespoon of apple cider vinegar

- 1 Tablespoon of hot pepper sauce;
- 2 Tablespoons of raw honey
- 1 Minced garlic clove
- 2 Teaspoons of fresh, minced ginger
- ½ Teaspoon of Chinese five Spice
- 1 Teaspoon of crushed red pepper flakes
- ¼ Cup of potato starch
- 2 Tablespoons of coconut oil
- 1 Pinch of sea salt
- 1 Pinch of freshly ground black pepper

Directions:

1. Into a medium deep bowl, mix the apple cider vinegar with the coconut aminos, the hot pepper sauce, the garlic, the honey, the ginger, the red pepper flakes and the Chinese five spices.
2. In another bowl; mix the starch with the chicken and season the mixture very well with a little bit of salt and 1 pinch of ground, black pepper.
3. Heat the coconut oil in a non-stick skillet and over a medium-high heat
4. When the oil melts, toss in the chicken and sauté it until it becomes brown for about 5 minutes
5. Add the chilies; then sauté for 2 additional minutes
6. When the chicken is perfectly cooked, add the sauce and stir your ingredients very well together
7. Let your ingredients boil for about 3 minutes
8. Serve and enjoy!

Nutritional information

- Calories per serving – 111.1 calories

- Fat per serving – 2 grams
- Saturated Fats – 0.5 gram
- Total Carbs per serving –2.1 grams
- Protein per serving – 21 grams

CHICKEN WITH ROSEMARY AND RED POTATOES

- ***Cooking Time: 55 minutes***
- ***Preparation Time: 15 minutes***
- ***Servings: 4***

- **NOTE:**

This recipe is very easy to male and doesn't need more than a few minutes; but it is very succulent with the flavorful taste of the lemon chunks. The addition of rosemary adds a special taste thanks to its anti-inflammatory proprieties.

INGREDIENTS

- 9 Pieces of chicken with the skin on and with the bone in
- 1 Pound of baby red potatoes
- ½ Of diced large onion
- 2 Sliced lemon
- 1 Juiced lemon
- 1/3 Cup of olive oil
- 2 Minced garlic cloves

- 1 Tablespoon of fresh rosemary
- Rosemary sprigs for garnishing
- ½ Teaspoon of crushed red pepper flakes
- 1 and ½ teaspoons of salt
- ½ Teaspoon of fresh ground pepper

Directions:

1. Preheat your oven to about 400 degrees F.
2. Grease a baking tray with cooking spray; then arrange the pieces of chicken with its side up in the tray
3. Arrange the potatoes, the sliced onion and the lemon slices in your tray
4. In a separate and small bowl; mix the lemon juice with the olive oil, the garlic, the rosemary, the crushed red pepper flakes, the salt and the pepper.
5. Pour in the mixture over the chicken and make sure your ingredients are very-well coated; then toss all the ingredients if needed
6. Sprinkle with a little bit of salt and 1 pinch of pepper
7. Bake your tray uncovered for around 1 hour or until the chicken and the potatoes are perfectly cooked.
8. Serve and enjoy your nutritious chicken meal.

Nutritional information

- Calories per serving – 230.1 calories
- Fat per serving – 11.5 grams
- Saturated Fat – 1.5 gram
- Total Carbs per serving – 1.21 grams
- Protein per serving – 27.2 grams

STUFFED CHICKEN WRAPPED WITH BACON

- ***Cooking Time: 50 minutes***
- ***Preparation Time: 10 minutes***
- ***Servings: 5***

- **NOTE:**

In addition to the creative idea of wrapping the chicken meat with bacon; you will like the stuffing made with the healthiest ingredients you can ever find with the artichoke hearts that help strengthen your nervous system. Not only this recipe will make you feel joyful with its delicious taste, but it will help you relax with the taste of chestnuts and its crispy texture underneath your teeth. You can grill your chicken or even bake it in the oven or make it in a skillet.

INGREDIENTS

- About 2 boneless and skinless chicken breasts
- ¼ Teaspoon of unrefined sea salt
- About 10 slices of organic and, especially, sugar-free bacon

- To prepare the stuffing
- 4 Chopped pieces of artichoke hearts
- ½ Cup of chopped and sliced water chestnuts
- ½ Cup of sun dried and finely chopped tomato
- ¼ Cup of pine nuts
- 1 Large, minced garlic clove
- 1 Teaspoon of fresh and finely chopped rosemary
- 1 Teaspoon of freshly ground black pepper
- ½ Teaspoon of smoked paprika

Directions:

1. First, start by preparing the stuffing by combining the ingredients altogether into a deep and small mixing bowl; then set it aside

2. Preheat your oven to about 375 degree Fahrenheit; then slice the chicken breasts into the middle; if you don't know how to do that; carefully follow the following instructions: put the blade of the knife into a parallel position with your cutting board; then place your hand in a flat position over the breast of chicken and slice

3. When you reach about ¾ of the way through the chicken meat, then stop and get ready to lay your chicken breasts over a cutting board; then with a meat mallet; gently pound your meat until you get the thickness of about ½ inch thickness

4. Put the flattened chicken breasts over your wooden cutting board and sprinkle with a little bit of salt and put about half of your stuffing into the middle of each of the chicken breasts

5. Evenly spread your stuffing over the chicken breast; but leave 1 inch around the stuffing

6. Tightly roll the chicken breasts with the strips of bacon

7. Put the chicken breasts with the side down, into a baking tray; then loosely cover the chicken with an aluminum

8. Bake your stuffed chicken breasts in your oven at about 375° F for about 40 minutes.

9. Remove the foil and drain the juice; then return your tray to the oven and cook it for about 20 minutes

10. Remove the tray from the oven; then remove let rest for about 10 minutes

11. Sliced the chicken breasts; then serve and enjoy!

Nutritional information

- Calories per serving –261.2 calories
- Fat per serving – 29.9 grams
- Saturated Fat – 0.59 gram
- Total Carbs per serving –14.8 grams
- Protein per serving – 60.6 grams

STUFFED CHICKEN WRAPPED WITH BACON

- ***Cooking Time: 15 minutes***
- ***Preparation Time: 5 minutes***
- ***Servings: 3***

- **NOTE:**

If you are following a Paleo Diet recipe and you want to eat something zesty and mouthwatering; then you won't find a recipe better than this one. The taste of the sauce, combined with the chicken breast will make you feel full and satisfied with these delicious ingredients.

INGREDIENTS

- 1 Pound of diced, boneless and skinless chicken breast (The cuts should be of about ¾ inches)
- ¼ Cup of almond flour
- 1 Cup of chicken stock
- ¼ Cup of raw honey
- ¼ Cup of coconut aminos

- ½ tablespoon of fresh peeled; then grated ginger
- 2 Grated garlic cloves
- 2 Teaspoon of coconut oil
- 2 Tablespoons of cooking oil
- 5 Cups of broccoli florets
- 1 Sliced, medium onion
- ¾ Pound of white sliced, button mushrooms

Directions

1. Start by trimming the chicken breast of fat; then pat it dry by using paper towels
2. In a bowl; mix the almond flour with the chicken breast and add the chicken breast; then remove the chicken to a dish
3. Now, prepare the sauce by mixing the flour with the chicken stock into a medium deep bowl
4. Add the honey, the coconut aminos, the grated ginger, the grated garlic and about 2 teaspoons of coconut oil; then stir very well until your ingredients become smooth
5. Set your ingredients aside
6. Place a large and non-stick wok over a medium heat and heat about 1 tablespoon of coconut oil in it
7. Once your oil is melted; then add the chicken pieces and evenly spread it
8. Sauté the chicken for about 5 minutes on each side; then remove the chicken from your wok and set it aside.
9. Add about 1 tablespoon of coconut oil to your wok and add the broccoli florets; the onions and the sliced mushrooms to the wok and sauté for about 4 minutes
10. Pour your sauce over the ingredients and let boil for about 2 minutes over a low heat; and keep stirring until your ingredients thicken

11. Season your ingredients with a little bit of salt and a little bit of pepper
12. Serve and enjoy!

Nutritional information

- Calories per serving –322 calories
- Fat per serving – 12.5 grams
- Saturated Fat – 2.4 gram
- Total Carbs per serving –26.3 grams
- Protein per serving – 28.3 grams

CHICKEN LEFTOVERS WITH FRESH SALAD

- ***Cooking Time: 35 minutes***
- ***Preparation Time: 5 minutes***
- ***Servings: 2-3***

- **NOTE:**

If you have leftovers of chicken meat at and you don't want to throw it; then this recipe is the best choice you can make. It is a nutritious meal with chicken meat and onion. It will make you feel full in a short time.

INGREDIENTS:

- 1 Pound of chicken breasts
- 12 Tablespoons of melted margarine
- 4 Tablespoons of grated onions
- 4 Pressed garlic cloves
- 4 Teaspoons of thyme
- 2 Teaspoons of salt
- 2 Teaspoons of pepper

- 2 Teaspoons of rosemary
- 1 Teaspoon of sage
- 1/2 Teaspoon of marjoram
- 4 Cooked and chopped leftover, chicken breasts
- 1/2 Cup of mayonnaise
- 1 Teaspoon of dill
- 1 Teaspoon of onion
- 1/2 Cup of chopped black olives

Directions

1. Start by mixing the margarine with the spices.
2. Coat the chicken with the mixture of the herbs
3. Put the chicken in a baking dish and bake it into a preheated oven for about 40 minutes to a heat of about 375 °F
4. To prepare the leftover chicken salad; mix the ingredients of the leftover and in a serving plate, put the lettuce; then serve your delicious meal

Nutritional information

- Calories per serving – 194.5 calories
- Fat per serving – 6.5 grams
- Saturated Fat – 1.1 gram
- Total Carbs per serving – 3.1 grams
- Protein per serving – 28.9 grams

CHICKEN CURRY WITH COCONUT

- ***Cooking Time: 45 minutes***
- ***Preparation Time: 5 minutes***
- ***Servings: 5***

- **NOTE:**

Chicken curry with coconut is a very- well balanced and flavorful dish with completely healthy ingredients that will make you feel full for the rest of the day. This is a very easy recipe to make; you will enjoy it!

INGREDIENTS

- 3 Diced and cut chicken breasts
- 1 Tablespoon of coconut oil
- 1 Cup of refrigerated coconut cream
- 1 Cup of chicken stock
- 2 Cups of diced carrots
- 1 Cup of chopped celery
- 2 Diced tomatoes

- 1 and ½ tablespoons of curry powder
- 1 Tablespoon of grated ginger
- ¼ Cup of roughly chopped cilantro
- 6 Minced garlic cloves
- 1 Pinch of salt
- 1 Pinch of pepper

Directions:

1. Start by sautéing the chicken into the coconut oil into a medium pot
2. When the outside of your chicken becomes white; add the cream of coconut; the chicken broth and combine your ingredients very well together
3. Add the celery, the carrots, and the tomatoes.
4. Add the curry powder and the ginger.
5. Cook your ingredients over a medium heat for about 40 minutes; make sure to stir from time to time
6. Add the garlic and the cilantro with 1 pinch of salt.
7. Cook your ingredients for about 5 minutes
8. Serve and enjoy your curry!

Nutritional information

- Calories per serving – 150.1 calories
- Fat per serving – 7 grams
- Saturated Fat – 2.5 gram
- Total Carbs per serving –8.1 grams
- Protein per serving – 15.9 grams

CHICKEN WITH CAJUN AND BLUEBERRIES

- ***Cooking Time: 40 minutes***
- ***Preparation Time: 10 minutes***
- ***Servings: 5-6***

- **NOTE:**

If you want to transform your ordinary chicken meat into a fancy meal with the mouthwatering taste of blueberry sauce; then go ahead and make this recipe. The taste of the fresh blueberries with the orange juice gives your dish a special and unique taste. And you are going to enjoy the crispy texture of the chicken.

INGREDIENTS

- 6 to 7 bones in and skin on chicken thighs
- 2 Tablespoons of Cajun seasoning
- 2 Cups of fresh blueberries
- ½ Cup of orange juice
- 1 Tablespoon of chili powder

- 1 Tablespoon of cinnamon powder
- 1 Cup of homemade BBQ sauce
- 1 Pinch of sea salt
- 1 Pinch of ground black pepper

Directions

1. Preheat your oven to a medium heat.
2. Season the chicken meat with the seasoning of the Cajun.
3. Put the blueberries, the orange juice, the chili powder, and the cinnamon into a blender.
4. Pulse your ingredients until it is very- well combined.
5. Pour the BBQ sauce over the ingredients and season it very well to taste; then pulse it again until it is very-well blended.
6. Refrigerate your sauce until it is ready to use.
7. Grill your chicken thighs over a high heat until it becomes brown on both its sides for about 2 to 3 minutes per each side.
8. Transfer your ingredients to an indirect source of heat; then cover your it and cook for about 30 minutes
9. Baste your chicken with BBQ blueberry sauce; then grill it over a direct heat or until your sauce caramelizes.
10. Set the chicken aside to rest for about 4 to 5 minutes
11. Serve and enjoy!

Nutritional information

- Calories per serving −339.4 calories
- Fat per serving − 15.5 grams

- Saturated Fat – 2.2 gram
- Total Carbs per serving –20.9 grams
- Protein per serving – 29.9 grams

CHICKEN WITH ALMOND

- ***Cooking Time: 25 minutes***
- ***Preparation Time: 4 minutes***
- ***Servings: 4***

- **NOTE:**

Do you miss enjoying the crispy texture of chicken with the almond flour and with the spicy taste of paprika? If yes, then this recipe is yours, you can enjoy this chicken recipe for lunch and you can make it in the oven or the grill. It is a very easy to make-dish too; you will love it.

INGREDIENTS

- 1 Pound of boneless and skinless chicken breasts, boneless, skinless
- ¾ Cup of almond flour
- ¼ Cup of arrowroot powder
- 1 Teaspoon of paprika
- 1 Teaspoon of cumin

- ½ Teaspoon of garlic powder
- ¼ Teaspoon of cayenne pepper
- 1 Teaspoon of black pepper
- 1 Teaspoon of sea salt
- 3 Lightly beaten white of egg
- 1 Tablespoon of olive oil to grease the rack with

Directions:

1. Preheat your oven to about 375° F.
2. Now, grease a rack of wire with a little bit of olive oil; then put a baking sheet lined with a foil paper
3. Cut the chicken breast meat into strips; around 2 inches each
4. Line three different bowls; then put the arrowroot into one bowl, the egg whites into another bowl
5. Put the almond flour, the paprika, the garlic powder, the cumin, the cayenne, the black pepper and the salt into a third bowl.
6. Now, dredge the chicken pieces into the whites of eggs
7. Dredge the chicken meat into the mixture of the almond flour and put it over a greased wire rack
8. Repeat the same process with the remaining ingredients
9. Bake your chicken for about 20 to 25 minutes or until it becomes golden
10. Serve and enjoy your dish!

Nutritional information

- Calories per serving –286.4 calories
- Fat per serving – 7.9 grams
- Saturated Fat – 0.8 gram
- Total Carbs per serving –10.3 grams
- Protein per serving – 41.3 grams

CHICKEN WITH ORANGE JUICE

- ***Cooking Time: 30 minutes***
- ***Preparation Time: 5 minutes***
- ***Servings: 3***

- **NOTE:**

What do you want more than the freshness of orange with the spicy taste of garlic powder? You can serve this dish with broccoli rice or any vegetables and fruits. This recipe makes a light and very unique recipe that you will like.

INGREDIENTS

- 3 Chicken breasts with the skin and the bone in
- For the marinade
- 2 cups of frozen concentrate orange juice
- ½ cup of soy sauce
- 1 Tablespoon of garlic powder
- 1 Pinch of Spice rub
- 1 Teaspoon of your favorite poultry spice rub

Directions:

1. Start by rinsing and removing the skin of the chicken; then put it a plastic bag and set it aside
2. Mix the ingredients of the marinade altogether; then pour your marinade over the breasts of the chicken into the plastic bag
3. Remove any excess of air; then tightly seal it
4. Put the marinade in the refrigerator for about 7 hours
5. Now, time for smoking your chicken
6. Prepare the smoker and let it stabilize at about 250° F.
7. Pour off any excess of the marinade from the chicken meat and discard it.
8. Rub the surfaces of your chicken with the rub of the spice
9. Put the chicken breasts into the smoker for 1 and ½ hours
10. Serve and enjoy!

Nutritional information

- Calories per serving –243.1 calories
- Fat per serving – 2.2 grams
- Saturated Fat – 0.4 gram
- Total Carbs per serving –26.3 grams
- Protein per serving – 29.2 grams

CHICKEN TERIYAKI WITH COCONUT AMINOS

- ***Cooking Time: 35 minutes***
- ***Preparation Time: 10 minutes***
- ***Servings: 3***

- **NOTE:**

This is an easy Teriyaki Chicken Recipe that won't take so much time for you to make. Chicken teriyaki makes a simple dish and a quick dinner too; you will love it.

INGREDIENTS

- 6 to 7 chicken legs
- ½ Cup of coconut aminos
- ½ Cup of raw honey
- ¼ Cup of fresh orange juice
- 2 Tablespoons of rice vinegar
- 1 Teaspoon of arrowroot flour
- 1 Tablespoon of fresh grated ginger

- About 2 minced garlic cloves
- 1 Teaspoon of sesame oil
- 1 Pinch of red pepper flakes
- For garnishing: sesame seeds and chopped green onions

Directions

1. Preheat your oven to about 425°F
2. Combine your ingredients, except for the chicken, in a large pot or saucepan over a medium heat
3. When the mixture starts boiling, stir your ingredients very well.
4. Remove the pot from the heat and season your raw chicken with a pinch of salt and 1 pinch of pepper
5. Grease a medium baking tray; then put the chicken chunks into the tray; then brush the chicken with the teriyaki sauce on all its sides. You can save a little quantity of the teriyaki sauce to use it later
6. Bake your chicken into the oven for about 25 minutes; then baste with the chicken with the mixture for about 5 minutes.
7. Make sure to flip the chicken pieces through the process of cooking.
8. When your chicken is perfectly cooked and the inner temperature reaches about 165° F; then you can broil the chicken for about 2 to 3 minutes
9. Remove the chicken from the oven; then brush it with the remaining quantity of the teriyaki sauce
10. Garnish the chicken with the green onions and the sesame seeds; then serve and enjoy with veggies.

Nutritional information

- Calories per serving – 130 calories

- Fat per serving – 4.6 grams
- Saturated Fat – 1.6 gram
- Total Carbs per serving –5.1 grams
- Protein per serving – 18.1 grams

GREEK STYLE BAKED CHICKEN

- ***Cooking Time: 45 minutes***
- ***Preparation Time: 15 minutes***
- ***Servings: 4***

- **NOTE:**

This Greek style recipe is very tender and succulent; it is also rich in exotic flavorful taste. You will be surprised with how scrumptious this recipe is and you will be addicted to it.

INGREDIENTS:

- 4 Tablespoons of coconut oil
- 4 Tablespoons of fresh lemon juice
- 3 Minced garlic cloves
- 1 Teaspoon of ground coriander
- ¼ Teaspoon of ground cumin
- 1 Teaspoon of sweet paprika
- 1/8 Teaspoon of chili powder
- ½ Tablespoon of salt

- ½ Teaspoon of ground black pepper
- ½ Bunch of fresh parsley
- ½ Bunch of fresh cilantro
- 4 Boneless and skinless chicken breasts

Directions:

1. Put all your ingredients into a food processor; but don't add the parsley, the cilantro, the parsley and the chicken.
2. Pulse your marinade about 5 times in order to finely mince your garlic.
3. The next step; add in the cilantro and the parsley; then pulse the ingredients for a several times.
4. Pulse your ingredients until it becomes very-well chopped
5. Slice your chicken into the half lengthwise in order to come up with about 8 thin chicken pieces
6. Pour your marinade over the chicken and toss it altogether; then set it aside for about 4 hours
7. Bake your chicken in the oven for about 40 minutes at a temperature of about 375° F
8. Remove the chicken from the oven; and serve with tzatziki sauce
9. Enjoy your dish!

Nutritional information

- Calories per serving –271.7 calories
- Fat per serving – 4.2 grams
- Saturated Fat – 0.8 gram
- Total Carbs per serving –41 grams
- Protein per serving – 21.4 grams

CHICKEN WITH PISTACHIO CRUST

- ***Cooking Time: 30 minutes***
- ***Preparation Time: 5 minutes***
- ***Servings: 2-3***

- **NOTE:**

Do you want to enjoy the taste of pistachios with baked chicken breasts? If yes, then this recipe is yours, with the ingredients packed with the crusty pistachios. Besides, this recipe is very practical and easy to make. You are going to enjoy this delicious chicken recipe.

INGREDIENTS:

- About 3 large chicken breasts
- 2 Beaten eggs
- 2 Tablespoons of stone ground mustard
- 1 Cup of finely chopped unsalted pistachios
- ½ Teaspoon of garlic powder
- ½ Teaspoon of onion powder
- ¼ Teaspoon of salt

Directions

1. Start by pounding the chicken breasts until it becomes of around ¾ inch thickness
2. In a deep and medium bowl; whisk your eggs; then add in the ground, stone mustard
3. Over a plate, combine altogether the crushed pistachios with the garlic, the onion powder and the salt; then mix very well until it is very-well blended
4. Dip the breast of chicken into the mixture of the egg; then coat the chicken with the crust of the pistachios. Repeat the same process with the other side
5. Place your chicken over a roasting rack. Then bake your ingredients at about 350°F for about 30 minutes.
6. Serve and enjoy your chicken with a salad of your choice!

Nutritional information

- Calories per serving –336 calories
- Fat per serving – 13 grams
- Saturated Fat – 1.8 gram
- Total Carbs per serving –23.2 grams
- Protein per serving – 31.9 grams

GRILLED CHICKEN WITH BROCCOLINI

- ***Cooking Time: 25 minutes***
- ***Preparation Time: 10 minutes***
- ***Servings: 3***

- **NOTE:**

This Chicken recipe with Broccolini and sauce is very delicious and it will surprise you with how delicious it will be. You can serve this recipe with charred Broccolini and it only takes a few minutes to do that. This recipe is gluten-free and completely healthy for all people to eat it.

INGREDIENTS:

- ½ Teaspoon of sea salt
- ½ Teaspoon of fresh cracked pepper
- ½ Teaspoon of Spanish paprika
- ⅛ Teaspoon of cayenne powder
- About 2 chicken legs with the bone in.
- 2 Teaspoons of coconut oil

- 1 Cup of Broccolini
- 1 Teaspoon of neutral flavored oil
- Chili flakes for garnishing and lemon wedges
- To prepare the Chimichurri:
- ¾ Cup of parsley
- 2 Tablespoons of olive oil
- 1 Tablespoon of cider vinegar
- 2 Minced garlic cloves
- ¼ Teaspoon of oregano
- ¼ Teaspoon of chili flakes
- ¼ Teaspoon of sea salt
- 1 splash of water

Directions

1. Preheat a BBQ to a medium-low heat.

In a small and deep bowl, combine altogether the fresh cracked pepper with the sea salt, the fresh cracked pepper, the paprika and the optional cayenne.

1. Drizzle about ½ teaspoon of the olive oil over both sides of each of the chicken legs.
2. Put the chicken legs over the BBQ skin with the side up; then bake it for about 15 minutes
3. Flip the chicken over the other side and cook it for 5 more minutes; put the Broccolini into a medium bowl and after that toss it with the sea salt; then cook for about 10 minutes
4. Meanwhile; prepare the sauce of chimchurri by blending all the ingredients together in a blender for about 2 minutes
5. Serve the chicken with the Broccolini and serve it with the lemon wedges and with chili flakes right on top.

Nutritional information

- Calories per serving – 363 calories
- Fat per serving – 23 grams
- Saturated Fat – 3.5 gram
- Total Carbs per serving – 17 grams
- Protein per serving – 18.9 grams

RECIPE 15: CHICKEN WITH COCONUT MILK

- ***Cooking Time: 3 hours***
- ***Preparation Time: 20 minutes***
- ***Servings: 5-6***

- **NOTE:**

You want to bake a meal with milk, but you don't know which type of coconut milk is the best to use; then this recipe is the best you can choose. This recipe made of braised chicken with coconut milk is the best you can choose. You are going to enjoy this easy recipe.

INGREDIENTS

- 3 Pounds of chicken breast
- 4 Tablespoons of coconut oil
- 1 Tablespoon of finely chopped lemongrass
- 1 Teaspoon of fine sea salt
- 1 Teaspoon of finely minced ginger
- 2 Cups of unsweetened coconut milk
- 2 Leaves of lime

- The zest of 1 lime
- 1 Red chili
- 5 Crushed garlic cloves
- 4 Slices of ginger
- 7 stems of cilantro
- ½ Cup of chopped Thai basil

Directions

1. Preheat your oven to about 325° F.
2. Start by melting the coconut oil over a medium-high heat into an oven steel tray or a heat proof pan.
3. Mix the lemon grass with the sea salt and the ginger into a bowl; then add 1 tablespoon of the coconut oil and mix the ingredients very well
4. If your chicken is tied up; then remove the string.
5. With the help of your hands, try separating the skin from your meat
6. Spread the rub of salt underneath the skin of the chicken.
7. Put the chicken in the saucepan; then sauté it until it becomes brown on all of its sides
8. Flip the chicken meat into the saucepan pot and brown it on all sides. Cook the chicken for about 10 minutes
9. Pour out most of your coconut oil; then pour in the coconut milk, the lime leaves, the lime zest, the chili, the garlic, the ginger and the cilantro.
10. Put your chicken back in the pan with the breast side up and cover your pot; then transfer to a preheated oven.
11. Braise your chicken for about 2 hours
12. Serve and enjoy!

Nutritional information

- Calories per serving – 147.5 calories

- Fat per serving – 6.8 grams
- Saturated Fat – 3.2 gram
- Total Carbs per serving – 10.1 grams
- Protein per serving – 12.8 grams

- **NOTE:**

If you liked our Paleo Chicken recipes, feel free to discover a wide range of our chicken books. You can find a diverse set of air fryer chicken recipes and other choices that you will enjoy reading and most importantly, you will enjoy making the recipes with simple ingredients.

CHAPTER 8

BEEF RECIPES

BEEF ROAST WITH COCOA

- ***Cooking Time: 25 minutes***
- ***Preparation Time: 5 minutes***
- ***Servings: 3***

- **NOTE:**

THIS RECIPE IS unique with the use of cocoa rub in it; it is a great choice for you to change the flavor. The taste of cumin and its combination with onion and chili powder adds an excellent taste to your dish. Enjoy this hearty and scrumptious meal you can ever try.

INGREDIENTS

- 2 Grass fed beef roast
- 1 Teaspoon of chipotle Chile powder
- ½ Teaspoon of onion powder
- ¼ Teaspoon of cumin
- ½ Teaspoon of kosher salt
- 1 Teaspoon of cocoa powder

Directions

1. Preheat your oven to about 325 degrees Fahrenheit and mix altogether your dry ingredients with the spice rub.
2. Trim your roast of any excess of fat
3. Generously coat your roast with the spicy cocoa rub.
4. Roast your ingredients for about 15 minutes at about 325 degrees Fahrenheit, then lower the heat to about 225° F and bake it for about 3 hours.
5. Your beef should be of about 150° F when you remove it from your oven
6. Let the beef meat be baked for about 145°F as internal temperature before you pull the beef meat from the oven and let it rest for about 10 minutes.
7. Serve and enjoy your delicious meal!

Nutritional information

- Calories per serving –251.9 calories
- Fat per serving – 9.9 grams
- Saturated Fat – 4 gram
- Total Carbs per serving –1.1 grams
- Protein per serving – 36.9 grams

Recipe 12: Beef Steak with orange juice
(Cooking Time: 20 minutes \ Preparation Time: 50 minutes \ Servings: 4-5)

- **NOTE:**

Discover this luxurious meal made of beef and of crispy orange beef. Enjoy the taste of the orange zest with the crispy texture of the arrowroot starch. You will never forget the taste of this recipe once you try it, so what are you waiting for; go ahead and enjoy your recipe.

INGREDIENTS:

- 2 Pounds of sirloin steak
- 2 Tablespoons of coconut aminos
- 1/3 Cup of arrowroot starch
- 1 Cup of coconut oil

The ingredients for the sauce

- 2 Tablespoons of arrowroot or cornstarch
- 1/3 Cup of fresh orange juice
- 3 Tablespoons of molasses
- 1 Tablespoon of rice vinegar
- 3 Minced garlic cloves
- 1 Teaspoon of minced fresh ginger
- ¼ Cup of thinly sliced orange rind
- ¼ Cup of finely chopped green onion

Directions:

1. Cut the meat into pieces of the same size
2. Add the coconut aminos to the pieces of meat pieces and toss the ingredients altogether.
3. Add in the arrowroot starch and coat your meat pieces very well
4. Put a wire rack in a cookie tray; then spread the pieces of meat into 1 single layer and set it aside to rest for about 40 minutes
5. When you only have about 10 minutes left before removing the meat from the freezer; pour the oil into a large non-stick wok.

6. Let the oil heat for about 5 minutes
7. Prepare a bowl and line it with a paper towel; then start frying the meat and cook it until it becomes golden for around 3 minutes per side.
8. Line a bowl with a paper towel and start frying meat
9. Remove the pieces of meat to the paper towel; then keep frying the remaining quantity until all of your meat is done.
10. Now, time to prepare the sauce of orange by mixing about 2 tablespoons of the arrowroot or the cornstarch with 1/3 cup of fresh orange juice, 3 tablespoons of molasses, 1 tablespoon of rice vinegar, 3 minced garlic cloves, about 1 teaspoon of fresh ginger, ¼ cup of minced thinly sliced orange rind and ¼ cup of finely chopped green onion.
11. Combine all of your sauce ingredients into a small and deep saucepan, then whisk and let the sauce boil for about 2 to 3 minutes

Nutritional information

- Calories per serving –216.8 calories
- Fat per serving – 9.6 grams
- Saturated Fat – 3.7 gram
- Total Carbs per serving –7.3 grams
- Protein per serving – 23.8 grams

CABBAGE ROLLS WITH GROUND BEEF

- ***Cooking Time: 40 minutes***
- ***Preparation Time: 25 minutes***
- ***Servings: 8-9***

- **NOTE:**

Have you ever thought that there could be another use for cabbage other than steaming it and making a supper with it? Get ready to learn a new and innovative, cabbage recipe. These cabbage rolls with the ground beef is very healthy and will help you lose weight in a short period of time. Besides, this recipe is scrumptious and irresistible.

INGREDIENTS

- 6 Tablespoons of coconut oil
- 1 Finely chopped onion
- 6 Minced garlic cloves
- 1 Pound of ground beef
- 1 Teaspoon of sea salt

- 1 and ½ teaspoons of black pepper
- 1 Teaspoon of dried dill
- 1 Teaspoon of mustard powder
- 2 Cups of cauliflower rice
- 2 Shredded carrots
- 1 head green cabbage
- 1 Can of tomato sauce

Directions:

1. Heat about 2 tablespoons of the coconut oil over a medium heat in a pan
2. Toss in the onion and sauté your ingredients until it becomes softened for about 6 minutes. Add in the garlic and keep sautéing for 1 additional sauté minute
3. Add the beef meat with 1 teaspoon of pepper; a little bit of salt and dill and the powder of the mustard; then cook for about 7 minutes; make sure to stir from time to time
4. When the pink colour of the meat disappears, add the cauliflower rice with the carrots
5. Remove the pan from the heat and set it aside for about 6 minutes. Stir in the cooked rice and carrots, then remove from the heat and set aside as you prepare the cabbage.
6. Cut out the cores of your cabbage and put in a pot filled with water over a medium high heat
7. Press the cabbage down to the pan and let boil for about 5 minutes
8. Remove the cooked cabbage from the boiling water with 2 forks; then strain the cabbage into a colander for about 1 minute
9. Peel off the leaves of cabbage; then stop when the cabbage leaves start to get dry and hard Return the cabbage to the boiling water and repeat the same process with the rest of the ingredients

10. Heat the coconut oil in the a pot over a low heat; then pour in the tomato sauce and the pepper
11. Let the ingredients simmer while you start making the rolls
12. Put the cabbage leaves over a cutting board; then remove any excess of cabbage spine
13. Spoon a little bit of your filling into right the base of the leaf of cabbage; then roll it altogether
14. Preheat your oven to about 325° F
15. Put the cabbage rolls into a saucepan; then pour the tomato sauce on top
16. Bake your ingredients until it is perfectly cooked for about 40 minutes
17. Serve and enjoy your meal!

Nutritional information

- Calories per serving –240.2 calories
- Fat per serving – 11.8 grams
- Saturated Fat – 4.3 gram
- Total Carbs per serving –12.5 grams
- Protein per serving – 19.9 grams

PALEO BEEF WITH BROCCOLINI

- ***Cooking Time: 20 minutes***
- ***Preparation Time: 60 minutes***
- ***Servings: 2-3***

- **NOTE:**

Have you ever ordered a beef dish with Broccolini and coconut aminos? This is a Paleo beef recipe that you will enjoy its fascinating taste. You will enjoy the combination of the delicious and the healthy ingredients of this recipe.

INGREDIENTS

- 1 Pound of scotch fillet beef
- 1 Tablespoon of Shaoxing wine
- 1 Tablespoon of coconut aminos
- ¼ Teaspoon of coconut oil
- 1 Teaspoon of corn flour
- 1 Tablespoon of vegetable oil
- 1 Large, peeled and chopped onion

- 1 large finely cut garlic clove
- 1 Bunch of washed and chopped Broccolini
- 1 Cup of raw almonds
- Cooked cauliflower rice

Directions

1. Start by washing; then pat dry the meat and cut it into slices of about ½ cm each
2. Put the meat into a large and deep bowl; then add the Shaoxing wine, the coconut aminos, the coconut oil and the corn flour
3. Stir very well to combine the ingredients; then cover it and refrigerate your ingredients for about 1 hour
4. Once you are ready, heat a wok; then pour the oil in it.
5. Add the onion and cook it over a medium high heat for about 1 minute; keep stirring
6. Add the garlic and keep stirring while you cook for about 1 minute
7. Raise the heat to medium high; then add the beef and cook for 1 additional minute
8. Add the beef; then cook and stir for about 1 additional minute
9. When your beef meat is not completely cooked; remove it from the heat and set it aside.
10. Turn the heat on; then add the almonds and the Broccolini.
11. Stir very well to combine it; then cover it with a firm lid and turn the heat down to low
12. Set your meal aside to cool for about 2 minutes
13. Remove the lid and stir very well
14. Return the beef meat to the pan; then mix and combine your ingredients very well

15. Serve your meal immediately with the steamed cauliflower rice.
16. Enjoy your meal!

Nutritional information

- Calories per serving –207 calories
- Fat per serving – 9.4 grams
- Saturated Fat – 1.9 gram
- Total Carbs per serving –14.5 grams
- Protein per serving – 14.6 grams

GROUND BEEF WITH ZUCCHINI

- *Cooking Time: 18 minutes*
- *Preparation Time: 5 minutes*
- *Servings: 3-4*

- **NOTE:**

You will enjoy this versatile recipe that is made only with a few ingredients. And if you want to find the best way that will help you lose weight; then you should try this recipe made of zucchini. Indeed, zucchini is known for its ability to fight overweight. Besides, zucchini is very beneficial by providing the body with Vitamin C and the other vitamins and nutrients it needs.

INGREDIENTS:

- 3 Medium fresh, cut zucchini
- 1 Pound of lean ground beef
- 1/2 Chopped medium onion
- 2 Chopped garlic cloves
- 1 Cup of jarred salsa with onions, chilies and tomatoes

- 1 Teaspoon of ground cumin
- 1 Pinch of salt
- 1 Pinch of pepper

Directions

1. Brown the ground beef with the chopped onions, the chopped garlic, a little bit of salt and a little bit of pepper.
2. Cook your ingredients over a medium high heat for 9 minutes
3. Add the salsa with the cumin; then cover and let simmer over a low heat for about 10 minutes
4. Add the chunks of zucchini; then let cook for around 9 more minutes
5. Serve and enjoy your nutritious meal!

Nutritional information

- Calories per serving –243.2 calories
- Fat per serving – 11.2 grams
- Saturated Fat – 4.6 gram
- Total Carbs per serving –9.2 grams
- Protein per serving – 25.1 grams

BEEF STROGANOFF WITH ZUCCHINI NOODLES

- ***Cooking Time: 35 minutes***
- ***Preparation Time: 10 minutes***
- ***Servings: 4***

- **NOTE:**

Did you know that the history of Beef Stroganoff dates back to more than 150 years ago? In addition to its ancient history, beef Stroganoff is healthy to eat and when combined with mushrooms, you won't be able to resist its delicious taste. And this is not all; you can enjoy this delicious meal with the steamed zucchini noodles. If you include this recipe in your daily meal; believe me, you will lose weight in no time.

INGREDIENTS:

- 1 Pound of diced stew beef
- 3 Teaspoons of divided coconut oil
- ¼ Teaspoon of salt
- ¼ Teaspoon of pepper
- ¼ Teaspoon of garlic powder

- 1 Sliced medium onion
- 8 Oz of thickly sliced baby Portobello mushrooms
- 3 Crushed garlic cloves
- ½ Teaspoon of paprika
- ¼ Teaspoon of dried thyme
- ¼ Teaspoon of onion powder
- 2/3 Cup of beef broth
- ½ Cup of full fat coconut milk
- 1 Tablespoon of chopped parsley

Directions

1. Start by coating the beef meat with about ½ teaspoon of salt, 1 pinch of pepper, and 1 pinch of garlic powder.
2. Rub the meat with your hands; then set it aside for about 3 minutes; meanwhile, melt about 2 teaspoons of coconut oil into an electric pressure cooker over a high heat
3. Let the oil melt in order to get a nice color of the meat; then sauté the meat for about 3 minutes
4. Repeat the same process in batches and if needed, add a little bit more of the oil
5. Remove each of the beef batches of the browned beef to a separate bowl in order to retain the juices.
6. Add the onion, the mushrooms, and about ¼ teaspoon of salt to a saucepan; then stir very well and cook your ingredients for about 9 to 10 minutes
7. Put the meat back into the electric pressure cooker; then add the mushrooms and the onion
8. Add the paprika, the garlic, the thyme, and the onion powder; then stir your ingredients very well
9. Add the broth of the beef to your pressure cooker; then close the lid and let the ingredients boil for about 15 minutes

10. When the time is up, remove the pressure cooker from the heat and set it aside to naturally release the pressure

11. Remove the lid of the pressure cooker; then pour in the coconut milk and let simmer over a medium high heat for a few minutes

12. Serve your dish with zucchini noodles and garnish with a little bit of parsley

Nutritional information

- Calories per serving – 101.1 calories
- Fat per serving – 6.2 grams
- Saturated Fat – 3.5 gram
- Total Carbs per serving – 8.1 grams
- Protein per serving – 3 grams

BEEF FAJITAS

- ***Cooking Time: 15 minutes***
- ***Preparation Time: 60 minutes***
- ***Servings: 3-4***

- **NOTE:**

Do you miss tasting the classic taste of fajitas with beef meat? Don't miss it anymore and make your own fajitas at home, according to simple tips and with simple ingredients that you can find in every house. Feel free to top with veggies of your choice.

INGREDIENTS

To prepare the marinade:

- 6 Minced garlic cloves
- ¼ Cup of extra virgin olive oil
- ¼ Cup of coconut aminos
- 1 and ½ teaspoons of cumin
- 1 Teaspoon of chilli powder
- ¼ Cup of chopped cilantro

- The Juice and the zest of two limes
- To prepare the Fajitas
- 1 and ½ pounds of skirt steak
- 1 Pinch of sea salt
- 1 Pinch of black pepper
- 1 Sliced red bell pepper
- 1 Sliced yellow bell pepper
- 1 Sliced green bell pepper
- 1 Large, sliced onion
- 2 Stemmed and seeded jalapeños, stem and seeds removed, sliced into strips
- 2 Sliced avocados
- 1 Chopped beefsteak tomato
- ¼ Cup of finely chopped cilantro

Directions:

1. Combine all of your ingredients into a zip top plastic bag of 1 gallon size.
2. Put the skirt steak into the prepared bag; then remove any excess of excess air; then seal the bag and shake it or massage it
3. Put the steak bag in the refrigerator and let marinate for about 60 minutes
4. Heat a non-stick iron pan over a medium heat; then remove the steak from the refrigerator and from the bah; then season both its sides with a pinch of salt and a little bit of black pepper
5. Put the steak over the pan; then sear it for about 5 minutes
6. Flip your steak; then cook it for 5 additional minutes
7. Remove the steak from the wok; then put it over a cutting board and cover it with a foil

8. Scrape any excess of fats and add the onion, the jalapeños and the pepper.
9. Add your marinade; the same you used to sauté your meat in order to sauté the vegetables for about 5 minutes
10. Slice the steak and arrange it in a serving platter with the rest of your ingredients and veggies
11. Top your dish with the avocado slices, the chopped tomato, and the cilantro.
12. Serve and enjoy!

Nutritional information

- Calories per serving –339.4 calories
- Fat per serving – 15.4 grams
- Saturated Fat – 2.4 gram
- Total Carbs per serving –21.1 grams
- Protein per serving – 30.1 grams

EASY BEEF KABOBS

- ***Cooking Time: 30 minutes***
- ***Preparation Time: 20 minutes***
- ***Servings: 2-3***

- **NOTE:**

Get ready to taste the best beef kabob you can ever tryed! This recipe will teach you all that you need to know to prepare a delicious kabob meal in an exotic way. You will enjoy this dish and you can do it collectively with your friends and family.

INGREDIENTS

- 2 Cups of coconut milk
- 2 Pounds of ground beef
- 4 Teaspoons of fresh lemon juice
- 1 Large peeled, seeded and diced cucumber
- 2 Tablespoons of fresh minced mint
- 1 Teaspoon of salt

Directions:

1. Preheat your oven to about 375°F; then drain the onions and press it with a sieve.
2. Mix the onion with about ½ teaspoon of salt; then set it aside for about 15 minutes and remove any excess of water
3. Mix the onion with the ground beef, the garlic, the egg, the remaining salt, the pepper, the turmeric, and the paprika
4. Divide the mixture of the meat into rectangles of about 6" of length
5. You can use metal skewers too, by pressing them through the beef kabobs.
6. Or you can put the kabobs in a baking tray; then bake it in your oven for about 15 minutes
7. When the time is up, flip the kabobs; then bake it on the other side for about 13 minutes
8. Serve and enjoy your beef kabobs; fresh mint!

Nutritional information

- Calories per serving –272.1 calories
- Fat per serving – 16.9 grams
- Saturated Fat – 2.6 grams
- Total Carbs per serving –21.1 grams
- Protein per serving – 19.1 grams

STEAK WITH BALSAMIC VINEGAR

- ***Cooking Time: 10 minutes***
- ***Preparation Time: 5 minutes***
- ***Servings: 3***

- **NOTE:**

With the combination of a diversity of herbs and the juicy taste of the balsamic vinegar, you can make a luxurious lunch or dinner. This recipe is very unique and impressive; you will like it and you can share it with your friends too.

INGREDIENTS

- 1 Pound of flank steak
- ¼ Cup of balsamic vinegar
- ½ Cup of extra virgin olive oil
- ½ Tablespoon of dried oregano
- ¼ Tablespoon of dried rosemary
- 6 Pressed garlic cloves
- 1 Teaspoon of salt

- ½ Teaspoon of pepper

Directions:

1. Mix altogether the vinegar, the oil, and the seasonings into a bowl; then whisk very well
2. Cut the flank steak into strips of about 1 inch each
3. Put the flank steak in a large platter or in a zip lock bag.
4. Pour the marinade over the steak
5. Let the steak marinate for an overnight in the refrigerator and make sure to remove it before cooking it for about 20 minutes.
6. When the steak becomes warm; prepare your grill by heating it to medium and start searing the steak for about 4 to 5 minutes per side
7. Let the steak rest for about 5 minutes
8. Serve and enjoy!

Nutritional information

- Calories per serving –274.2 calories
- Fat per serving – 13.9 grams
- Saturated Fat – 4.3 grams
- Total Carbs per serving –14.9 grams
- Protein per serving – 23.0 grams

Recipe 20: Beef Lasagna with zucchini

(Cooking Time: 90 minutes \ Preparation Time: 30 minutes \ Servings: 4)

- **NOTE:**

Are you looking for a delicious lasagne, but you are afraid of gaining weight? If yes, then we have found the best solution for you, which is to try this beef lasagne with zucchini. The ingredients of this recipe are very-well chosen with great care. The addition of basil and fresh oregano adds a fresh taste that will make you enjoy the zucchini lasagne.

INGREDIENTS:

- 3 Medium zucchini
- 1 Tablespoon of salt
- 1 Pound of ground beef
- 1 and ½ teaspoons of ground black pepper
- 1 Green bell pepper
- 1 Chopped onion
- 1 Cup of tomato paste
- 1 Can of tomato sauce
- ¼ Cup of red wine
- 2 Tablespoons of chopped fresh basil
- 1 Tablespoon of chopped fresh oregano
- Boiling water
- 1 large egg
- 1 Container of low-fat ricotta cheese
- 2 Tablespoons of chopped fresh parsley
- 1 Package of drained and thawed frozen chopped spinach
- 1 Pound of fresh mushrooms

Directions:

1. Preheat your oven to about 325° F and grease a deep baking tray
2. Slice the zucchini in a lengthwise way into thin slices
3. Sprinkle the slices with a pinch of salt and set it aside to drain into a colander

4. To prepare the sauce, cook; then add the ground beef and the black pepper into a large skillet over a medium high heat and cook for about 5 minutes.

5. Add in the green pepper and the onion; then cook and stir until the meat becomes no longer pink. Add in the tomato paste, the tomato sauce, the wine, the basil, and the oregano

6. Let the ingredients boil; then reduce the heat and let the sauce simmer for about 19 minutes; stir from time to time.

7. In the meantime, combine the egg with the ricotta and the parsley into a deep bowl until your ingredients are very-well combined

8. Now, time to assemble the lasagna; and to do that spread about half of the sauce into the bottom of a prepared tray with the zucchini slices

9. Add about half the mixture of the ricotta; then add the spinach and the mushrooms

10. Repeat the same process when with the remaining sauce, the zucchini slices and the ricotta mixture.

11. Cover your ingredients with a foil paper; then bake it for about 45 minutes

12. Remove the foil; then raise the temperature of about 350 degrees F

13. Bake the lasagna for about more 15 minutes

14. Serve and enjoy your lasagna!

Nutritional information

- Calories per serving – 329 calories
- Fat per serving – 19.8 grams
- Saturated Fat – 3.8 grams
- Total Carbs per serving – 13.8 grams
- Protein per serving – 29 grams

- **NOTE:**

If you enjoyed our Paleo beef recipes, feel free to discover a wide range of our beef steak books. You can find a diverse set of air fryer beef recipes and other choices that you will enjoy reading and most importantly, you can cook according to the method you prefer.

CHAPTER 9

VEGAN RECIPES

VEGAN FALAFEL WITH ZUCCHINI

- ***Cooking Time: 40 minutes***
- ***Preparation Time: 10 minutes***
- ***Servings: 9***

- **NOTE:**

NOT ONLY IS this recipe very healthy and delicious; but it is completely vegan. This recipe is completely vegan and rich in anti-inflammatory ingredients. When you taste this recipe, you will get addicted to it and its delicious taste.

INGREDIENTS

- 2 Small rinsed, grated, organic zucchini
- 2 Cups of riced cauliflower
- 1 Cup of finely diced onion
- 2 Teaspoons of minced garlic
- 2 Teaspoons of dried cilantro
- 2 Teaspoons of dried parsley
- 2 Teaspoons of dried mint

- 1 and ½ teaspoons of cumin
- ½ Teaspoon of turmeric
- ½ Teaspoon of cayenne pepper
- The zest of 1 lemon
- 1/8 Teaspoon of black pepper
- 1 Teaspoon of sea salt
- 1 Cup of almond meal
- 1 Beaten egg
- ½ Teaspoon of baking soda
- ¼ Cup of coconut flour
- ¼ Cup of organic olive oil

Directions

1. Preheat your oven to about 375° F degrees
2. With a handheld grater; then grate the zucchini and remove any excess of water by squeezing it with a paper towel
3. Put the grated and the drained zucchini into a large and deep bowl
4. To rice the cauliflower; rinse the cauliflower; then cut it into small florets and put it in a food processor
5. Pulse the cauliflower into the texture of the size of rice
6. Add about 2 cups of the riced cauliflower to the zucchini, and stir it very well until it becomes evenly incorporated
7. For your vegetable mixture, add the onion, the garlic, the cilantro, the parsley, the mint, the cumin, the turmeric, the cayenne, the lemon zest, the salt, the pepper and stir very well
8. In a medium bowl, beat the egg and add in the baking soda
9. Add the egg mixture to a large bowl; then add 1 cup of almond meal or flour

10. Set the mixture aside to rest for several minutes; then add around ¼ cup of the coconut flour
11. Cover a large baking tray with a non stick aluminum foil; then spread a little amount of the olive oil over the foil
12. Now, form balls of medium size with your bare hands
13. Roll your ingredients into the coconut flour before putting it over the aluminum foil
14. With a silicone brush, brush the top of your falafel with a little bit of olive oil
15. Bake your ingredients for about 40 minutes in the oven; make sure to flip once or twice
16. Serve and enjoy!

Nutritional information

- Calories per serving –216 calories
- Fat per serving – 20.1 grams
- Saturated Fat – 2.9 grams
- Total Carbs per serving –8.1 grams
- Protein per serving – 4 grams

MUSHROOMS AND ZUCCHINI CASSEROLE

- ***Cooking Time: 3 minutes***
- ***Preparation Time: 3 minutes***
- ***Servings: 3***

- **NOTE:**

This is a very easy to make recipe with the delicious taste of sautéed Zucchini and the mushrooms. This recipe is easy to come together with its very simple ingredients and you can prepare it in a very short time.

INGREDIENTS

- 4 Tablespoons of ghee
- ½ Pound of quartered mushrooms
- ½ Teaspoon of Himalayan salt
- 1 Teaspoon of freshly cracked pepper
- 4 Chopped green onions
- 3 Minced garlic cloves
- 6 Medium, cut zucchinis

- 1 Tablespoon of magic mushroom powder
- ¼ Cup of fresh chopped parsley
- 3 Chili peppers

Directions:

1. Start by melting the ghee into a heavy skillet over a high heat.
2. Stir in the mushrooms; then sprinkle with a little bit of salt and pepper
3. Cook your ingredients until they become golden for a few minutes
4. Remove your ingredients to a bowl; then lower the heat and add in the garlic and the green onion
5. Cook your ingredients for around 2 to 3 minutes
6. Add the zucchinis; then return the mushrooms to your skillet
7. Add the peppers and garnish with parsley
8. Serve and enjoy your dish!

Nutritional information

- Calories per serving – 115 calories
- Fat per serving – 8.8 grams
- Saturated Fat – 5.2 grams
- Total Carbs per serving – 7.8 grams
- Protein per serving – 3.5 grams

RECIPE 23: CARROTS PASTA

- ***Cooking Time: 10 minutes***
- ***Preparation Time: 5 minutes***
- ***Servings: 2***

- **NOTE:**

Carrots pasta is your best recipe if you want to lose weight. In addition to its healthy ingredients; carrots pasta is packed with nutrients and it is light and delicious. You can enjoy carrots pasta for a light lunch or dinner.

INGREDIENTS

- 2 Tablespoons of olive oil
- 2 Tablespoons of onion or shallot
- 1 Cup of chopped mushrooms
- ¼ Teaspoon of sea salt
- ¾ Teaspoon of dried basil
- 1 Pinch of black pepper
- About 3 large carrot ribbons

- ¾ Cup of marinara sauce
- Chopped fresh parsley

Directions:

1. Start by heating the oil in large pan.
2. Add the onion or the shallot; then sauté for about 2 minutes.
3. Add the salt, the mushrooms, the basil, and the pepper
4. Cook your ingredients for about 6 minutes
5. Add the carrot ribbons and sauté for about 1 minute.
6. Pour in the sauce, and let your ingredients, cook for about 6 to 8 minutes or until the noodles are perfectly cooked
7. Top your dish with a little bit of parsley
8. Serve and enjoy your carrot pasta!

Nutritional information

- Calories per serving –242.1 calories
- Fat per serving – 10.3 grams
- Saturated Fat – 1.4 grams
- Total Carbs per serving –36.2 grams
- Protein per serving – 7.3 grams

ALMOND FLOUR PANCAKE

- ***Cooking Time: 20 minutes***
- ***Preparation Time: 5 minutes***
- ***Servings: 5-6***

- **NOTE:**

This is an awesome recipe for you if you want to taste a delicious and nutritious meal. You will enjoy making this recipe because it doesn't need more than simple ingredients. You can also serve these almond pancakes with mango or peach.

INGREDIENTS

- Oil for frying
- ½ Cup of Almond Flour
- ½ Cup of Tapioca Flour
- 1 Cup of Coconut Milk
- 1 Teaspoon of salt
- ½ Teaspoon of Kashmiri Chili Powder
- ¼ Teaspoon of Turmeric Powder

- ¼ Teaspoon of freshly ground black pepper
- ½ Chopped red onion
- 1 Handful of chopped cilantro leaves
- 1 Minced Serrano pepper
- ½ Inch of grated ginger

Directions:

1. To make the Batter:
2. In a large and deep bowl, mix the almond flour with the tapioca flour, the coconut milk and the spices altogether.
3. Then, stir in the onion, the cilantro, the Serrano pepper and the ginger.
4. Heat a non-stick wok over a low heat; then pour in the oil and let it heat for about 3 to 4 minutes
5. Pour about ¼ cup of the batter into your wok; then spread it in your wok
6. Fry your pancake for about 2 minutes per each side
7. Drizzle with a little bit more oil if needed
8. Repeat this process of the remaining quantity of batter and when you are done
9. Serve and enjoy your vegan dish with green chutney!

Nutritional information

- Calories per serving –97.4 calories
- Fat per serving – 7.3 grams
- Saturated Fat – 3.2 grams
- Total Carbs per serving –1.8 grams
- Protein per serving – 6.1 grams

SPINACH QUICHE

- ***Cooking Time: 35 minutes***
- ***Preparation Time: 10 minutes***
- ***Servings: 8***

- **NOTE:**

With this mini quiche, you are absolutely going to discover a new and delicious vegan recipe that you are going to enjoy so much. It is a recipe filled with nutrients and in healthy ingredients to come up with a great dish that you can have any time of the day or you can save it to enjoy it during the following day!

INGREDIENTS:

- 2 Cups of almond flour
- ½ Teaspoon of salt
- ¾ Teaspoon of baking soda
- ¾ Cup of melted coconut oil
- 1 and ½ tablespoons of water
- ½ Finely diced red onion

- 2 Minced garlic cloves
- 2 Handfuls of chopped baby spinach
- ½ Cup of sliced sun dried tomatoes
- ½ Cup of sliced and pitted red olives
- 4 Large organic eggs
- ¼ Cup of nutritional yeast
- 2 Tablespoons of coconut milk
- 1 Pinch of pepper

Directions:

1. Preheat your oven to about 350°F; then line a muffin tin with some muffin liners.
2. Whisk your ingredients altogether with the almond flour, the salt, and the baking soda.
3. Add about ½ cup of the melted coconut oil and about 1 and ½ tablespoons of water
4. Add more oil if needed; then press the pastry crust into a large ball
5. Press your pastry crust into the liners of the muffin tin
6. Poke holes into your quiche; then put it into the oven and bake it for about 15 minutes
7. While your crust is being cooked, sauté the onion into a frying pan over a medium heat for about 5 minutes
8. Add in the garlic and then sauté it until it becomes fragrant for about 2 minutes
9. Add spinach for about 5 minutes
10. Remove the pan from the heat and turn off the heat; then add in the dried tomatoes; then set it aside
11. In a medium bowl, whisk the eggs with the yeast, the milk and the pepper.
12. Once your quiche crust becomes gold, remove it from the heat; then spoon the mixture into your crust and top it with the mixture of the egg

13. Put your quiche into your oven and bake it for about 30 minutes
14. Serve and enjoy!

Nutritional information

- Calories per serving – 150 calories
- Fat per serving – 1.9 grams
- Saturated Fat – 5.9 grams
- Total Carbs per serving – 5.9 grams
- Protein per serving – 13.1 grams

TORTILLAS WITH THYME AND BEET

- ***Cooking Time: 25 minutes***
- ***Preparation Time: 10 minutes***
- ***Servings: 6***

- **NOTE:**

These vegan tortillas are very light and easy to make. It is rich in a diversity of flavours and it can give you a very unique flavour. You can enjoy this type of tortillas with any meal of your choice. These tortillas will help you lose weight in a very short period of time with salads.

INGREDIENTS

- 6 Tablespoons of warm water
- 2 Tablespoons of chia seeds
- 1 and ½ cups of grated beets
- 1 Cup of almond flour
- 1 Tablespoon of fresh thyme
- ¼ Teaspoon of salt

- 1 Tablespoon of olive oil

Directions:

1. Start by soaking the chia seeds into the warm water for about 10 minutes.
2. Preheat your oven to about 390°F; then grease a parchment paper and line it with a baking sheet.
3. In a large and deep mixing bowl, mix your ingredients altogether and gently mix in order to form a soft dough.
4. Mix the ingredients with your fingers until you obtain sticky dough
5. Divide your dough into about 6 equal parts.
6. Form balls from the parts and gently press it to flatten it
7. Arrange the flattened balls over the cookie sheet and gently press it into a shape of thin tortillas of a round form.
8. Repeat the same step for the remaining dough; then put the tortillas over the cookie sheet
9. Put the cookie sheet into the bottom rack of your oven and bake it for about 20 minutes
10. Serve your tortillas with toppings of your choice

Nutritional information

- Calories per serving –220 calories
- Fat per serving – 4.4 grams
- Saturated Fat – 0.0 grams
- Total Carbs per serving –35.1 grams
- Protein per serving – 6.1 grams

BROCCOLI BITES

- ***Cooking Time: 10 minutes***
- ***Preparation Time: 5 minutes***
- ***Servings: 12***

- **NOTE:**

Today, you can make these easy to make vegan, Paleo broccoli bites. The addition of cashews adds a special taste and enriches your dish. You will enjoy this broccoli recipe as a snack, a simple appetizer and even as a dinner. Broccoli is known for its anti-inflammatory effects too. So what are you waiting for, make your own broccoli bites.

INGREDIENTS

- 2 and ½ cups of organic raw broccoli pieces
- 2 and ½ cups of organic cashews
- ¼ Cup of organic onion
- 2 Cloves of freshly minced organic garlic
- 2 Tablespoons of extra-virgin olive oil
- About 1 organic jalapeno

- ¼ Cup of nutritional yeast
- ½ Teaspoon of Himalayan pink salt

Directions

1. Pulse the cashews and the broccoli pieces in a food processor and process it until you obtain small chopped pieces.
2. Add all of your remaining ingredients to your food processor and pulse it with the cashew and the broccoli pieces.
3. Pulse your ingredients until it is very well combined
4. Adjust the seasonings and squeeze about 1 spoon of the ingredients once a time until you shape the size of balls from the paste
5. Place your balls over a dehydrator tray; then dehydrate it at about 115° F for about 4 hours; you can also bake your broccoli bites on a cookie sheet for about 12 minutes in the oven.
6. Refrigerate the balls in the refrigerator for about 10 minutes
7. Serve and enjoy your broccoli balls!

Nutritional information

- Calories per serving –201 calories
- Fat per serving – 12.1 grams
- Saturated Fat – 2.6 grams
- Total Carbs per serving –13.2 grams
- Protein per serving – 11.8 grams

ONION SALAD

- ***Cooking Time: 5 minutes***
- ***Preparation Time: 3 minutes***
- ***Servings: 2-3***

- **NOTE:**

This onion salad is really great and easy to make. You can add other ingredients of your choice. You can add tomatoes and green peppers. It is a fresh salad that will make a great dinner if you don't want to cook.

INGREDIENTS:

- 1 Small, sliced red onion
- 2 Peeled and sliced cucumbers
- 3 Medium juiced limes
- 2 Tablespoons of chopped cilantro
- 1 and ½ tablespoons of olive oil
- 1 Pinch of salt
- 1 Pinch of black pepper

- Finely chopped parsley leaves

Directions

1. Put the onions in a large bowl and sprinkle a little bit of salt over it
2. Rub the onion with the salt; then cover it with water and set it aside for about 5 minutes
3. Drain the onions; then rinse it very well
4. Put the sliced onions, the sliced cucumbers, the lime juice, the chopped cilantro, and the olive oil into a large bowl.
5. Mix very well; then taste and add a little bit of salt as needed.
6. Garnish with the parsley
7. Serve your salad your salad immediately and enjoy it!

Nutritional information

- Calories per serving – 152.2calories
- Fat per serving – 13.8 grams
- Saturated Fat – 1.8 grams
- Total Carbs per serving –7.2 grams
- Protein per serving – 1.3 grams

PUDDING WITH AVOCADO

- ***Cooking Time: 10 minutes***
- ***Preparation Time: 5 minutes***
- ***Servings: 2***

- **NOTE:**

You can't find a simpler pudding recipe than this one. This pudding is made with avocado and topped with crispy pistachios. There is absolutely no question that this pudding is healthy and will make you feel full.

INGREDIENTS

- 1 Ripe, de-pitted and peeled ripe avocado
- ¼ Cup of soaked pistachios into warm water for about 15 minutes
- 5 tbsp water or coconut water
- 1 Pinch of salt
- 1 Teaspoon of pure vanilla extract
- 1 Teaspoon of rose water

- ½ Teaspoon of almond extract
- 1 Teaspoon of lemon juice
- Salt and finely chopped pistachios

Directions:

1. Put all of your ingredients, except for the garnish into a food processor or a power blender
2. Once your mixture becomes smooth, transfer your pudding into about 2 small jars
3. Cover the ingredients and refrigerator for around 30 minutes
4. When you are ready to serve your pudding; then garnish with a little bit more of pistachios
5. Serve and enjoy your pudding!

Nutritional information

- Calories per serving –231.1 calories
- Fat per serving – 8.6 grams
- Saturated Fat – 2.1 grams
- Total Carbs per serving –25.6 grams
- Protein per serving – 3 grams

CREPE WITH ARROWROOT FLOUR

- ***Cooking Time: 10 minutes***
- ***Preparation Time: 15 minutes***
- ***Servings: 3***

- **NOTE:**

Making arrowroot crepes is a fantastic way to prepare a balanced breakfast that is rich in proteins. You can try this crepe with arrowroot with vegetables and fruits. Besides, arrowroot is known for being used in the primitive cultures; this type of flour was used in healing some wounds, especially poisonous wounds.

INGREDIENTS:

- 5 Large eggs
- ½ Cup of blanched almond flour
- 2 Tablespoons of arrowroot flour
- 2 Tablespoons of water
- 2 Teaspoons of honey
- 1 Teaspoon of pure vanilla extract

- 1 Pinch of unrefined sea salt
- A little bit of coconut oil

Directions:

1. Beat your eggs with a little bit of salt into a large bowl. Add the honey and the vanilla.
2. Make sure not to leave any lumps and refrigerate your batter for around 15 minutes
3. Heat a non stick medium cast iron wok or pan over a medium heat; then brush it with a little bit of coconut oil.
4. If your pan is very well-seasoned; then brush with a little bit of coconut oil as long as you need.
5. Pour about ¼ cup of your batter into a pan; then swirl it into the tilt; then spread it
6. Let the crepe cook for about 40 seconds
7. Spread the crepe with the spatula before it thickens, then flip it and cook it o the other side for about 15 seconds
8. Remove the crepe to a platter; then stir the batter between the crepes
9. Repeat the same process with the rest of your batter
10. Arrange your crepes one on top of the other; then serve it with fruits
11. Serve and enjoy your crepe!

Nutritional information

- Calories per serving –302 calories
- Fat per serving –23.1 grams
- Saturated Fat – 2.8 grams
- Total Carbs per serving –19.5 grams
- Protein per serving – 8.5 grams
- **NOTE:**

If you are interested in learning more about our Vegan Recipes, you will find a wide range of options and books to enjoy. So please, don't hesitate to download it and share it you're your friends. You will find completely vegan recipes that you will love and you won't even miss the taste of meat with our vegan recipes.

CHAPTER7: VEGETARIAN RECIPES

FRIED BROCCOLI FLORETS

- ***Cooking Time: 15 minutes***
- ***Preparation Time: 10 minutes***
- ***Servings: 5-6***

- **NOTE:**

If you want a simple and very delicious dish that you want to enjoy with low calories; then you should try this cauliflower recipe, not only it is nutritious; but it doesn't need more than a few minutes to make.

INGREDIENTS

- 1 large and cut head of cauliflower; make sure the cauliflower florets are quite small
- 2 Large eggs
- To coat the cauliflower florets:
- ¼ Cup of almond meal or ground almonds
- ¼ Cup of tapioca flour
- 2 Tablespoons of coconut flour
- 1 Teaspoon of garlic powder

- 1 Teaspoon of onion powder
- 1 Teaspoon of paprika powder
- 1 Teaspoon of coriander powder
- 1 ½ Teaspoons of salt
- ½ Teaspoon of black pepper
- To prepare the red sauce:
- 1 Tablespoon of olive oil
- 1 Finely grated garlic clove
- 1 Tablespoon of tomato paste
- The juice of ½ Lime
- 1 Teaspoon of honey
- 1 Pinch of salt
- 1 Pinch of chili flakes or powder

Directions

1. Preheat your oven to about 430° F.
2. Now, prepare the cauliflower; then in a small bowl; whisk the eggs and set it aside.
3. Whisk all of the ingredients into a deep bowl and mix very well
4. Line a baking tray with a non stick parchment paper; then grease it with a little bout of coconut oil
5. Dip each of the cauliflower florets into the mixture if the egg and remove any excess of egg
6. Coat your ingredients with the crumbly mixture
7. Once you have finished with all the quantity of the cauliflower florets; place the tray into the middle shelf of the oven.
8. Set the timer to about 12 minutes and the temperature to about 390°F; in the meantime; prepare your red sauce by mixing all of its ingredients into one pan and cook it over a high heat.

9. When the sauce starts boiling, lower the heat and keep stirring for one additional minute
10. Remove the sauce from the heat and set it aside
11. Transfer the cauliflower florets to a serving platter; then drizzle with a little bit of sauce
12. Serve your cauliflower with the sauce
13. Enjoy this delicious dish!

Nutritional information

- Calories per serving – 109.9calories
- Fat per serving – 5.1 grams
- Saturated Fat – 0.8 grams
- Total Carbs per serving – 14.5 grams
- Protein per serving – 5.4 grams

CAULIFLOWER RISOTTO

- ***Cooking Time: 20 minutes***
- ***Preparation Time: 15 minutes***
- ***Servings: 3***

- **NOTE:**

If you have chosen to follow a Paleo diet and you are frustrated that you will miss eating risotto; then this cauliflower risotto is a recipe that you should try as soon as possible. The ingredients of this recipe are cheap and easy to find in any house. You will like the texture of this recipe; it is really irresistible.

INGREDIENTS

- 2 Cups of finely diced cauliflower
- ¾ Cup of finely diced carrots
- 1 Cup of finely diced zucchini
- ½ Finely diced medium onion
- 2 Large minced garlic cloves
- 3 Tablespoons of olive oil

- 1 Cup of dry white wine
- 2 Cups of vegetable stock
- 1 Heaped teaspoon of arrowroot flour combined with about 1/5 cup of hot water
- 1 Tablespoon of coconut oil
- 1 Cup of grated Parmesan cheese
- To make the macadamia burnt butter: use about 10 macadamia nuts and smashed t into little crumbs; then add to it about 2 tablespoons of organic butter+ ½ minced garlic clove and 1 pinch of salt

Directions:

1. Cut the onion and the garlic; then put the Macadamia nuts into a plastic bag; then lay it over a cutting board underneath a tea towel; then smack it with a rolling pin until your nuts are totally crushed into very little chunks and into small crumbs.
2. Grate the cheese and set it aside; then heat up a frying wok over a medium heat
3. Sauté the onion into about 3 tablespoons of extra virgin olive oil over a medium heat for about 5 minutes
4. Add the garlic and cook it for about 5 minutes; then stir from time to time
5. Rice the cauliflower, the zucchini and the carrots into tiny cubes
6. After about 10 minutes of cooking add the wine to your frying wok with the onion and the garlic; then let the ingredients boil over a high heat for about 2 to 3 minutes
7. Pour in about 2 cups of stock to the base of the risotto; then stir and cooker for about 4 minutes over a medium heat; meanwhile, add the macadamia crumbs to your second pot; then toast it over a high heat for about 2 minutes

8. Make sure to stir every few seconds in order to prevent any burning
9. Once the butter is ready, set it aside and add about 2 cups of the vegetable stock to the risotto base; the stir and cook your ingredients for about 4 minutes over a medium heat.
10. Set the butter aside to dissolve for 2 minutes; then set it aside
11. Add the flour water mixture to the risotto and stir very well
12. Add the cauliflower and the carrots first; then cook for about 1 to 2 minutes
13. Add the zucchini with 1 tablespoon of butter and add the Parmesan cheese; then cook and stir altogether for about 2 minutes
14. Garnish with the macadamia butter and season with the ground black pepper
15. Serve and enjoy!

Nutritional information

- Calories per serving – 107.8 calories
- Fat per serving – 5.5 grams
- Saturated Fat – 1.6 grams
- Total Carbs per serving – 9.2 grams
- Protein per serving – 5.7 grams

SOUP WITH CAULIFLOWER AND GARLIC

- ***Cooking Time: 20 minutes***
- ***Preparation Time: 10 minutes***
- ***Servings: 5***

- **NOTE:**

This simple cauliflower soup is made with chopped cauliflower. It is very smooth and light; you will enjoy it so much with a set of flavorful ingredients.

INGREDIENTS

- 1 Tablespoon of ghee
- 1 Medium chopped white onion
- 1 Cored and roughly chopped cauliflower head
- 3 Chopped garlic cloves
- 3 Cups of vegetable stock
- ⅔ Teaspoon of sea salt
- ½ Teaspoon of ground black pepper
- ¾ Cup of diced bacon

- 1 Large egg
- Coconut oil for frying

Directions:

1. Heat about 1 tablespoon of the ghee until it becomes hot
2. Sauté the onion for about 3 minutes or until it becomes soft
3. Add the garlic, the cauliflower and the stock; then bring the ingredients to boil
4. Season your ingredients with a little bit of salt and with 1 pinch of ground black pepper
5. Turn off the heat and cook it for about 8 to 10 minutes
6. Fry the bacon until it becomes crispy for about 8 minutes
7. Add the egg into small pan or in a metallic bowl; and whisk in this egg for around 3 minutes
8. Transfer the cauliflower soup ingredients to a processor and process it for a couple of minutes
9. With a hand held blender, add in the egg cream
10. Garnish with the fresh herbs, the chives, the parsley and the bacon
11. Serve and enjoy!

Nutritional information

- Calories per serving – 176.9 calories
- Fat per serving – 11.5 grams
- Saturated Fat – 9.6 grams
- Total Carbs per serving – 15.6 grams
- Protein per serving – 5.6 grams

BEETROOT COUSCOUS

- ***Cooking Time: 15 minutes***
- ***Preparation Time: 10 minutes***
- ***Servings: 2-3***

- **NOTE:**

This beetroot couscous is derived from a vegetable recipe that is based on mint, walnuts and a few delicious ingredients. You will enjoy this healthy and nutritious recipe and you can serve it without worrying about how many calories it has.

INGREDIENTS

- ⅔ Cup of hazelnuts
- 1 Medium, finely diced brown onion
- 1 Tablespoon of coconut oil
- ½ Teaspoon of sea salt
- 2 Medium, peeled and diced raw beetroots
- 2 Finely minced garlic cloves
- 1 Teaspoon of ghee

- 1 Cauliflower, broken into small florets
- 2 Tablespoons of chopped parsley or mint
- For garnishing:
- 1 Tablespoon of lemon zest
- The Juice of ⅔ medium lemon
- 1 Tablespoon of Balsamic vinegar
- 3 Tablespoons of hazelnut oil
- 1 Tablespoon of extra-virgin olive oil
- ½ Teaspoon of sea salt
- ½ Teaspoon of pepper
- ½ Teaspoon of Dijon mustard
- ½ Teaspoon of honey
- ½ Teaspoon of sesame oil

Directions

1. Start by heating a frying pan and toast the hazelnuts over a medium heat for about 2 to 3 minutes.
2. Stir the ingredients frequently in order to prevent any burning.
3. Transfer the ingredients to a medium bowl; then set it aside to cool a little bit.
4. Place the ingredients in a towel and rub it together with both your hands
5. Sauté the onion in a little bit of ghee and add a pinch of salt
6. Put the beetroot, the garlic and the hazelnuts into a food processor; then grind the ingredients into very small crumbs
7. Finely chop the nuts with the help of a knife
8. Add the ground beetroot, the garlic and the hazelnuts to the sautéed onion; then cook altogether for about 1 or 2 minutes
9. Add a little bit of ghee if needed; then put the cauliflower

florets into your food processor; then grind altogether into very small crumbs.

10. Add the ingredients to the beetroot mixture; then stir very well and transfer your ingredients to a large bowl

11. Mix the ingredients very well; then add the dressing over the salad and add the parsley or the mint and stir very well altogether.

12. Adjust the taste of the salt; then add a little bit of lemon juice

13. Garnish with the whole hazelnuts, the parsley and a little bit more of grated lemon zest.

Nutritional information

- Calories per serving –219.6 calories
- Fat per serving –4.01 grams
- Saturated Fat – 0.4 grams
- Total Carbs per serving –39 grams
- Protein per serving – 5.5 grams

SALAD WITH ZUCCHINI AND MINT LEAVES

- ***Cooking Time: 15 minutes***
- ***Preparation Time: 10 minutes***
- ***Servings: 2-3***

- **NOTE:**

What is better than tasting a light salad with zucchini and mint? It is a refreshing salad that you will enjoy anytime with any dish. Feel free to add toppings of your choice.

INGREDIENTS

- 4 Grated carrots
- 1 and ½ teaspoons of coriander seeds
- ½ Teaspoon of ground cumin or seeds
- 2 Tablespoons of apple cider vinegar
- ½ Teaspoon of sea salt
- 4 Tablespoons of olive oil
- ½ Deseeded and finely cut Red chili
- About 10 Mint leaves

Directions:

1. Mix the vinegar, the salt and the pepper into a large bowl and set it aside.
2. Heat a wok and over a medium heat; then cook the coriander and the cumin seeds without oil for about 2 minutes; but don't forget to keep stirring in order to prevent any burning
3. Grind the toasted coriander and the cumin seeds with a mortar or in a grinder; then put the spices in a frying pan and mix very well
4. Add the carrots and the chili; then stir in the dressing of the vinegar
5. Add the oil and mix very well
6. Now, cut the mint into fine cuts and mix it with the grated carrots before serving it
7. Serve and enjoy with garnish of mint!

Nutritional information

- Calories per serving – 166.1 calories
- Fat per serving – 11 grams
- Saturated Fat – 2.3 grams
- Total Carbs per serving – 39 grams
- Protein per serving – 5.5 grams

Recipe 36: Baked Vegetables

(Cooking Time: 40 minutes \ Preparation Time: 10 minutes \ Servings: 4)

- **NOTE:**

The vegetable mixture in this recipe is baked to make a perfect dish. Celery plays a vital role in providing the body with vitamins and important nutrients for the body. The zucchini is also a great source of healthy components.

INGREDIENTS

- 4 Tablespoons of coconut oil
- 4 Chopped stalks of celery
- 2 and ½ cups of vegetable broth
- 2 Chopped sweet potatoes
- 3 Sliced carrots
- 4 Sliced parsnips
- 2 Small, chopped zucchini
- 4 Minced garlic cloves
- 2 Chopped onions
- 5 Chopped baby Portobello mushrooms
- 3 Finely, chopped rosemary sprigs
- 1 Pinch of ground sea salt
- 1 Pinch of ground black pepper

Directions

1. Preheat your oven to about 375°F.
2. Now, heat the coconut oil into a large frying wok over a medium heat
3. Start by cooking the celery, the sweet potatoes the carrots, the parsnips, the zucchini, about 1 onion and the garlic.
4. If you need a little bit more of coconut oil, don't hesitate to add a little bit more
5. Remove the ingredients from the pan; then add it to a casserole pan
6. Add the onion, the chopped mushrooms and the garlic
7. Add the rosemary and stir very well.

8. When your onions start getting soft, then add the stock and let the ingredients boil for about 3 minutes
9. Remove the liquid from the heat and slowly add the mixture over the pan
10. Season your ingredients very well with black pepper
11. Bake your ingredients in a baking tray in an oven for about 30 minutes
12. Serve and enjoy!

Nutritional information

- Calories per serving – 164 calories
- Fat per serving – 3.8 grams
- Saturated Fat – 0.4 grams
- Total Carbs per serving – 31.6 grams
- Protein per serving – 2.6 grams

SPINACH DIP

- *Cooking Time: 5 minutes*
- *Preparation Time: 10 minutes*
- *Servings: 2*

- **NOTE:**

If you want a fantastic dish with very few and affordable ingredients, then you should try this spinach dip. The addition of oil adds a special and unique taste to this recipe; you are going to like it.

INGREDIENTS

- 2 Cups of tightly packed, defrosted spinach
- 1 Tablespoon of coconut oil
- 2 Tablespoons of extra virgin olive oil
- 1 Large and thinly sliced brown onion
- ⅔ Teaspoon of sea salt
- 2 Finely diced, large garlic cloves
- 1 Teaspoon of mild curry powder
- ½ Cup of coconut cream

- 1 Tablespoon of lemon juice

Directions

1. Defrost the spinach; then put the frozen spinach balls or the blocks into a medium bowl with a little bit of hot water for about ½ an hour to 1 hour.
2. Strain; then squeeze any excess of liquid
3. Heat a medium frying pan over a medium-high heat; then add the coconut oil let the ingredients simmer over a low heat.
4. Add the salt and the onion; then sauté your ingredients for about 6 minutes and stir
5. Add the spinach; the garlic and the curry; the, stir for around 1 to minutes
6. Add the coconut cream with the lemon juice and stir very well for 1 additional minute until
7. Combine all of your ingredients together; then season with the salt and pepper
8. Serve and enjoy with one of our chicken recipes or beef recipes!

Nutritional information

- Calories per serving – 157 calories
- Fat per serving – 13.3 grams
- Saturated Fat – 3.2 grams
- Total Carbs per serving – 4.9 grams
- Protein per serving – 5.7 grams

Recipe 37: Soup with vegetables

(Cooking Time: 18 minutes \ Preparation Time: 5 minutes \ Servings: 3)

- **NOTE:**

If you want to enjoy a soup full of nutritious ingredients, then this recipe is yours. The use of squash adds a special taste to this recipe and helps improving the circulation of blood within the body. You can use this recipe as a snack, a simple dinner or even as an appetizer.

INGREDIENTS

- 3 Quartered and cut, medium yellow squashes
- 2 Small diced red onions
- 2 Cups of shredded carrots
- 2 Cups of frozen peas
- 6 Chopped garlic cloves garlic
- 1 and ½ cups of veggie broth
- The juice of 2 lemons
- 2 Teaspoons of lemon
- 1 Tablespoon of herbs de Provence
- 1 Tablespoon of organic butter
- 1 Pinch of sea salt
- 1 Pinch of pepper

Directions:

1. In a large saucepan and over a medium heat, melt the butter
2. Add the chopped onions, the garlic and the shredded carrots; then sauté for about 4 minutes
3. Add the diced yellow squash, the herbs de Provence, the sea salt and the pepper to taste.
4. Stir in the veggies; then add the veggie broth
5. Cover your ingredients and let it simmer for about 18 minutes
6. Remove the pan from the heat; then add the lemon juice,

the lemon zest, the peas and adjust the seasonings with a
little bit of salt and 1 pinch of ground black pepper
7. Serve and enjoy your dish!

Nutritional information

- Calories per serving – 140.3 calories
- Fat per serving – 6.2 grams
- Saturated Fat – 3.1 grams
- Total Carbs per serving – 15.3 grams
- Protein per serving – 6.8 grams

FRUIT BOWL

- ***Cooking Time: 5 minutes***
- ***Preparation Time: 5 minutes***
- ***Servings: 4***

- **NOTE:**

Make sure to make this Paleo bowl because it is simple, light and tasty. Fruits bowl is rich in nutrients and vitamins; you can't miss enjoying this fruit bowl no matter what.

INGREDIENTS:

- 1 Packet of organic unsweetened Acai
- 1 and ¼ cups of frozen mixed berries
- 1 Medium or Small frozen banana
- ½ Cup of unsweetened almond milk
- 1 Heaping tablespoon of cashew butter
- 1 Tablespoon of honey
- 2 Tablespoons of chia seeds
- 2 Tablespoons of collagen peptides

- 1 Tablespoon of coconut oil
- For the Toppings
- Use bee pollen for the topping
- Use cacao nibs to top your ingredients
- Coconut flakes; unsweetened
- Fresh fruits to top with

Directions:

1. Combine all of your ingredients into a high speed blender; then blend it over a medium heat for about 1 minute
2. Make sure that all of your ingredients are very well blended
3. Pour the obtained mixture into a large bowl; then top with the cacao nibs, the coconut flakes and toppings of your choice
4. Serve and enjoy!

Nutritional information

- Calories per serving –449 calories
- Fat per serving –19 grams
- Saturated Fat –9 grams
- Total Carbs per serving –45 grams
- Protein per serving – 21 grams

COFFEE SMOOTHIE

- ***Cooking Time: 5 minutes***
- ***Preparation Time: 10 minutes***
- ***Servings: 2***

- **NOTE:**

Do you want to enjoy a delicious smoothie coffee with completely health ingredients? With simple ingredients and in a very short time; you can prepare a very delicious coffee that will make you feel fresh and start a great day!

INGREDIENTS

- ½ Cup of chilled, brewed coffee
- 1 Cup of coconut milk or almond milk
- 1 Tablespoon of almond butter
- 1 Teaspoon of pure vanilla extract
- 2 Tablespoons of chocolate protein powder
- 1 Tablespoon of cocoa powder
- 1 Tablespoon of maple syrup

- ¼ to ½ cup of chia seeds

Directions:

1. Blend your ingredients altogether except for the chia seeds
2. Put your ingredients altogether into a reseal able jar; then add the seeds of chia
3. Make sure that your jar is sealed very well
4. Refrigerate the jar in the refrigerator for about 3 hours
5. Shake the frit bowl; then serve and enjoy!

Nutritional information

- Calories per serving – 186calories
- Fat per serving – 16 grams
- Saturated Fat – 5.9 grams
- Total Carbs per serving – 8.1 grams
- Protein per serving – 2.1 grams

BANANA SMOOTHIE

- *Cooking Time: 5 minutes*
- *Preparation Time: 5 minutes*
- *Servings: 2*

- **NOTE:**

If you want a different and creative smoothie for an overnight; then you should try this one. You can add any other types of fruits to your taste; it is a refreshing and delicious smoothie that you will enjoy anytime of the day and it is very good to drink at night too because of its calming effects over our body.

INGRDIENTS:

- 1 Cup of berries
- 1 Sliced banana
- 2 Tablespoons of walnuts
- 2 Teaspoons of chia seeds
- 2 Teaspoons of hemp seeds
- ¼ Cup of almond milk or coconut milk

Directions:

1. Start by peeling and cleaning all of your ingredients in a bowl
2. Mix your ingredients and sprinkle it with seeds
3. Add in the milk
4. Serve and enjoy your delicious smoothie

Nutritional information

- Calories per serving – 136.7 calories
- Fat per serving – 3.1 grams
- Saturated Fat – 0.4 grams
- Total Carbs per serving – 29.3 grams
- Protein per serving – 7.5 grams

CHAPTER 10

FISH AND SEAFOOD RECIPES

SHRIMP AND VEGETABLE SALAD

- ***Cooking Time: 5 minutes***
- ***Preparation Time: 5 minutes***
- ***Servings: 2***

- **NOTE:**

THIS IS A VERY easy shrimp salad that combines very healthy ingredients. Shrimp salad is rich in proteins and in zesty lemon juice; it is great for a very simple dinner. You can top it with fruits and ingredients of your choice.

INGREDIENTS:

- 1 Pound of cooked shrimp
- 2 Cups of diced watermelon
- 1 Cup of cherry or halved grape tomatoes
- ¼ Cup of olive oil
- 1 medium of juiced lime
- 1 Tablespoon of chopped fresh mint
- 1 Tablespoon of chopped, fresh parsley

- 1/8 Teaspoon of sea salt
- 1/8 Teaspoon of black pepper

Directions:

1. Mix the shrimp with the watermelon, and the tomatoes into a large bowl; then season your ingredients with 1 pinch of salt and 1 pinch of pepper.
2. In a covered jar, mix altogether the lime juice with the olive oil and the herbs
3. Season your ingredients with a pinch of black pepper
4. Toss your salad with the prepared dressing and set it aside to chill for a few minutes before serving it
5. Serve and enjoy your salad!

Nutritional information

- Calories per serving –194.1 calories
- Fat per serving –7.9 grams
- Saturated Fat –0.3 grams
- Total Carbs per serving –7 grams
- Protein per serving – 23 grams

FRIED TILAPIA

- ***Cooking Time: 10 minutes***
- ***Preparation Time: 5 minutes***
- ***Servings: 4-5***

- **NOTE:**

This delicious seasoned tilapia makes a light and delicious meal that you can enjoy with your family for a light dinner. Tilapia is packed with nutrients and vitamins. It is a very fast and easy to make dish.

INGREDIENTS

- 1 Pound of tilapia, diced into about strips of ½ inch each
- ½ Cup of coconut flour
- 1 Tablespoon of garlic powder
- 2 Teaspoons of salt
- 2 Teaspoons of cumin powder
- 1 Dash of pepper
- Coconut oil

- To prepare the white sauce
- ½ Cup of mayonnaise
- 1 Tablespoon of lime juice
- 1 Teaspoon of dried oregano
- ½ Teaspoon of cumin powder
- 1 Pinch of chili pepper
- ¼ Tablespoon of raw honey
- 5 lettuce leaves
- 1 Cup of salsa
- 2 Tablespoons of chopped cilantro
- 5 Slices of lime

Directions

1. Start by making the white sauce and mix all of your ingredients altogether with the help of a fork
2. Stir in the honey if your sauce is still very sour
3. To prepare the fish; mix altogether the coconut flour, the garlic powder, the cumin powder and the salt, pepper in a large bowl
4. Put the fish strips into a medium bowl; then coat with the mixture of the coconut flour
5. Now, heat the coconut oil in a large or a medium pan; then add the fish strips to the coconut oil and fry it for a few minutes
6. Repeat the same process with the rest of the ingredients
7. Transfer the fried fish to a paper towel
8. Serve and enjoy!

Nutritional information

- Calories per serving – 165.1 calories
- Fat per serving – 2.1 grams

- Saturated Fat –0.0 grams
- Total Carbs per serving – 11 grams
- Protein per serving – 22.9 grams

FISH MINI CAKES

- ***Cooking Time: 5 minutes***
- ***Preparation Time: 6 minutes***
- ***Servings: 5-6***

- **NOTE:**

Fish Mini cakes are rich in protein; you will enjoy tasting these salmon cakes and you can serve it with salads or any other dips. These mini cakes also help in improving the memory and in providing the body with necessary nutrients.

Ingredients

- 1 Can of Boneless and Skinless drained Salmon
- ½ Peeled and chopped onion
- 1 1/2 Tablespoon Coconut Flour
- 2 Large beaten eggs
- 1 Rib of diced celery
- 1 Tablespoon of dried dill
- 1 Teaspoon of lemon pepper

- ¼ Teaspoon of sea Salt
- 3 Tablespoons of coconut oil

Directions

1. In a large and deep bowl, shred salmon fish with the help of a fork; then add the cut onion, the celery and the spices
2. Sift in the coconut flour and mix very well
3. Crack in the eggs and whisk very well until your ingredients become very well incorporated
4. Add the eggs to the mixture and combine the ingredients very well together; meanwhile, heat the coconut oil into a large wok
5. Shape your batter into about 5 to patties
6. Gradually, add the patties to the pan; then cook it until all the sides of the patties are golden
7. Let the patties rest for about 3 minutes; then serve and enjoy!

Nutritional information

- Calories per serving –198.7 calories
- Fat per serving –9.3 grams
- Saturated Fat –2.8 grams
- Total Carbs per serving –2.9 grams
- Protein per serving – 24.3 grams

Recipe 44: Fish Curry with coconut milk
(Cooking Time: 5 minutes \ Preparation Time: 6 minutes \ Servings: 5-6)

- **NOTE:**

This curry recipe is not only a perfect fish curry, but it is also very satisfying and surprising with its extraordinary nutrients and with the vitamins it provides. The addition of chopped red pepper with ginger adds a natural spicy taste you will like, for sure.

INGREDIENTS

- 2 Tablespoons of light olive oil
- 1 Chopped onion
- ½ Chopped red pepper
- ½ Chopped green pepper
- 1 Fresh, finely chopped chili
- 3 Crushed garlic cloves
- 1 Finely chopped fresh ginger root
- 4 Tablespoons of curry paste
- 1 Can of coconut milk
- 1 Pound of cut, white fish fillet
- 1 Pinch of freshly ground black pepper
- A little bit of fresh coriander

Directions:

1. Start by heating the ghee into a saucepan; then fry the pepper; the onion and the chili over a medium heat for about 12 minutes
2. Add the minced garlic and the ginger and fry it all for about 1 minute
3. Add the curry and keep stir frying for about 2 minutes
4. Add a drizzle of lemon juice
5. Pour in the coconut milk and stir very well; then let simmer for about 5 minutes.
6. Add the fillets of the fish and season it with a little bit of black pepper; then cook for about 4 minutes
7. Top with coriander; then serve and enjoy your curry!

Nutritional information

- Calories per serving –207 calories
- Fat per serving –8.2 grams
- Saturated Fat –5.7 grams
- Total Carbs per serving –6.4 grams
- Protein per serving – 22.2 grams

FRIED SALMON WITH CAPERS

- ***Cooking Time: 10 minutes***
- ***Preparation Time: 5 minutes***
- ***Servings: 4***

- **NOTE:**

Whether you are on a gluten free-diet, you are following a sugar-free diet or you are adopting the Paleo diet; then this recipe will suit you all. It is very simple with simple ingredients and easy steps; it won't take more than a few minutes for you to prepare this recipe.

INGREDIENTS

- 2 Tablespoons of coconut oil
- 6 Salmon fillets or you can choose any type of white fish
- 1 Pinch of salt to taste
- 1 Pinch of ground black pepper
- 1 Thinly sliced small onion
- 1 Thinly sliced Anaheim Chili

- 3 Thinly sliced garlic cloves
- 2 Bay leaves
- ½ Teaspoon of chopped oregano
- 2 Cups of crushed tomatoes
- ¼ Cup of Green Olives
- 2 Tablespoons of Capers
- Lime wedges to serve

Directions:

1. Pour the oil onto a large skillet over a medium high heat
2. Generously season the fish with a pinch of salt and a pinch of pepper and press it with your fingers
3. Now, add the fish to the seasoned fish to the hot skillet and cook it until it becomes golden into its bottom for about 4 minutes
4. Make sure to flip the fish from one side to the other and cook it for about 2 minutes over the other side.
5. Remove the fish from the pan; then carefully put it on the platter
6. Add the chili and the onion; then sauté for about 3 minutes
7. Add in the garlic and sauté for about 30 seconds.
8. Add in the oregano, the bay leaves, the crushed tomatoes, the green olives, and the capers.
9. Let the ingredients simmer for about 5 minutes and cook until your ingredients become thick
10. Put the fish again in the pan and let your ingredients simmer for about 3 minutes
11. Remove the bay leaves
12. Serve your dish with the lime wedges

Nutritional information

- Calories per serving –275.9calories
- Fat per serving – 14.1 grams
- Saturated Fat –2.2 grams
- Total Carbs per serving –0.9 grams
- Protein per serving – 34.6 grams

SHRIMP WITH CHIMCHURRI

- *Cooking Time: 7 minutes*
- *Preparation Time: 3 minutes*
- *Servings: 3*

- **NOTE:**

A Zesty and very fast, flavorful recipe for the Chimichurri Shrimp, with a zesty ingredients; this recipe is very unique with the cilantro chimichurri sauce! It is a very simple recipe to make; fast and nutritious.

INGREDIENTS

- 1 Pound of large peeled raw prawns, deveined
- 2 Teaspoons of olive oil
- To prepare the Chimichurri Sauce:
- 1 Bunch of Cilantro
- 1 Bunch of Italian Parsley
- ¼ Cup of fresh lime juice
- ½ Cup of olive oil

- ¼ Cup of chopped onion
- 2 Minced garlic cloves
- 1 Pinch of salt
- ¾ Teaspoon of kosher
- ½ Teaspoon of smoked paprika

Directions:

1. Heat the oil into a large skillet over a medium high heat; then add the shrimp and sauté it for about 5 minutes.
2. Lower the heat and put the garlic and the onion in a food processor; then pulse the ingredients for a 1 or two minutes
3. Add the parsley and pulse your ingredients again
4. Add the oil, Turn heat down to medium low.
5. Add the oil, the lime juice, the smoked paprika and the salt; then pulse until all of your ingredients are very well combined.
6. Set your ingredients aside into small serving bowl.
7. When the shrimp is perfectly cooked, toss it with about half of the sauce of the chimichurri.
8. Serve and enjoy with a salad!

Nutritional information

- Calories per serving –230.2 calories
- Fat per serving –16.2 grams
- Saturated Fat –4.5 grams
- Total Carbs per serving –8.4 grams
- Protein per serving – 18.1 grams

SALMON JERKY WITH SRIRACHA

- ***Cooking Time: 7 minutes***
- ***Preparation Time: 3 minutes***
- ***Servings: 3***

- **NOTE:**

Tis Jerky Spice Salmon is filled with sweet and hot ingredients. It is very healthy and perfect for a seafood Paleo dinner. You will like the taste of this recipe that is rich in vitamins and nutrients. It will also boost your metabolic system.

INGREDIENTS

- 3 Trimmed scallions with the roots removed
- 3 Cups of ice water
- 4 Teaspoons of honey
- 2 Teaspoons of Sriracha hot sauce
- 4 Teaspoons of cider vinegar
- 3 Teaspoons of avocado oil
- 2 Teaspoons of flax seed oil

- 1 Teaspoon of kosher salt
- 1 Pound of salmon filet with the skin removed
- 1 and ½ teaspoons of Jamaican Jerk seasoning
- 4 Cups of baby arugula
- 2 Cups of julienned and cut finely chopped cabbage
- 2 Cups of julienne cut radish
- ¼ Cup of toasted pepitas

Directions:

1. Cut the scallion into two inches of length; then cut it lengthwise into thin strips.
2. Submerge the scallion strips into icy water; then set it aside.
3. Stir in the honey and the sriracha into a small dish; then combine it very well.
4. Remove 2 teaspoons of honey and put it into a large mixing bowl; then add the vinegar, about 2 teaspoons of canola oil, the flax oil and about ½ teaspoon of salt
5. Whisk your ingredients very well together and mix it to combine the ingredients
6. Sprinkle about ½ teaspoon of salt over the salmon fish; then season the Jerk
7. Heat about 1 teaspoons of canola oil into a large and heavy skillet over a medium high heat
8. Add the salmon with the skinned-side in the up position; then cook until your ingredients become crispy and brown right into the bottom for about 5 minutes
9. Flip the salmon over, then remove it from the skillet and cook for 4 minutes.
10. Now, time to prepare the salad by adding the cabbage to the salad turnips or the daikon, the radishes and the arugula to a large bowl with your dressing; then toss very well to coat.

11. Serve your salmon with the mixture of honey sriracha
12. Drain your scallions and top your dishes with it
13. Serve and enjoy!

Nutritional information

- Calories per serving –80.2 calories
- Fat per serving –1 grams
- Saturated Fat –0.0 grams
- Total Carbs per serving –2.1 grams
- Protein per serving – 16 grams

SOUP WITH MUSSELS

- ***Cooking Time: 15 minutes***
- ***Preparation Time: 5 minutes***
- ***Servings: 6-7***

- **NOTE:**

Mussels are not only a great source of protein, but it is very practical to make on a busy night. You can try this soup with any other side dish or main dish. So what is better than enjoying a Paleo seafood dish packed with nutrients? You will never regret making this recipe.

INGREDIENTS:

- 1 Tablespoon of coconut oil
- 1 Small cut onion
- 1 Large handful of fresh parsley
- 3 Garlic cloves
- 1 Teaspoon of crushed red pepper flakes
- ½ Cup of dry white wine
- 1 Can crushed tomatoes

- 1 Can of diced tomatoes
- 2 Cups of vegetable broth
- ½ Teaspoon of salt
- 2 Pounds of fresh live mussels

DIRECTIONS:

1. Start by heating the coconut oil into a large baking tray over a medium heat
2. Chop the onion and peel it; then add it to the skillet
3. Cut the parsley and set it aside; then crush the garlic cloves and cut the onion; then add it to your skillet
4. Finely chop the parsley; then add it to the garlic and the onion and stir
5. Let your ingredients cook for about 30 seconds; then pour in the wine and stir
6. Open up the cans of the tomatoes and add it to the pan with the vegetable broth, the parsley and the stir very well
7. Cover your ingredients, then increase the heat and cook your ingredients until it starts boiling
8. Lower the heat and let your ingredients simmer; meanwhile; remove the thread from the mussels and remove any barnacles
9. Put the mussels in a colander and then rinse it with the cold water.
10. Tap the mussels and if they remain open; discard it and add the mussels
11. Once your soup is still simmering, add the mussels to it; then cook until all of the mussels are open for about 10 to 15 minutes. If most of the mussels are open; then discard any mussel that remains closed
12. Pour the remaining parsley into bowls; then serve and enjoy!

Nutritional information

- Calories per serving –259.3 calories
- Fat per serving –5.6 grams
- Saturated Fat –1.0 grams
- Total Carbs per serving –13.1 grams
- Protein per serving – 30.2 grams

CARROT FISH CAKE

- ***Cooking Time: 40 minutes***
- ***Preparation Time: 10 minutes***
- ***Servings: 4***

- **NOTE:**

This recipe is rich in vitamins and packed with flavour. This fish pie is made with great care and with healthy ingredients like coconut milk instead of cream. All the ingredients of this recipe are low in fat and helps lowering the risk of having heart disease.

INGREDIENTS

- About 4 medium sized sweet potatoes
- 2 Tablespoons of coconut oil
- ¼ Cup of coconut milk
- ¼ Cup of coconut flakes
- 1 Pound of white fish; diced into small chunks
- 1 Can of coconut milk
- 1 Cup of chopped carrots

- ½ Cup of chopped green beans
- 1 Cup of chopped leek
- 2 Teaspoons of fresh grated ginger
- 1 Pinch of salt
- 1 Pinch of pepper
- 3 Boiled and chopped eggs

Directions:

1. Start by boiling the sweet potatoes for about 15 minutes
2. Peel the potatoes and process it with about 2 tablespoons of the coconut oil and with about ¼ cup of the coconut milk
3. Hard boil the 3 eggs
4. Pre-heat your oven to about 350°F.
5. Heat the remaining quantity of the coconut milk into a medium saucepan over a medium heat. When your ingredients start boiling, add in the chopped carrots, the leek, and the green beans.
6. Dice the fish into cubes of about 1 inch each; then add it to the pot.
7. Grate a little bit of ginger and add it to your; then season it with 1 pinch of pepper and cook your ingredients for a few additional minutes
8. Pour the mixture of the fish into a medium baking tray or in ramekins
9. Now peel the eggs; chop it and add it to the mixture of the fish
10. Spread the mashed mixture right on top of your fish mixture
11. Sprinkle a little bit of coconut flakes right on top of the mash of the potatoes
12. Put the baking tray in the oven for about 20 minutes

13. Remove the baking tray from the oven; then serve and enjoy it!

Nutritional information

- Calories per serving –359 calories
- Fat per serving –5.1 grams
- Saturated Fat –0.0 grams
- Total Carbs per serving –35.9 grams
- Protein per serving – 44 grams

HERBS-STUFFED FISH

- ***Cooking Time: 30 minutes***
- ***Preparation Time: 5 minutes***
- ***Servings: 4-5***

- **NOTE:**

The combination of white fish with herbs adds a special taste to this fish recipe. Not only herbed-stuffed fish will make you feel full in a short time; but it will also make ignite energy in your body, not to mention how tasty the herb stuffed fish is.

INGREDIENTS:

- 2 Pounds of large whitefish
- The juice of 1 lemon
- ¼ Cup of oil
- 1 Teaspoon of cayenne
- 1 Teaspoon of cumin

Directions:

- Heat the oven to about 350°F; then wash the fish and sprinkle a little bit of lemon.
- Let your ingredients stand aside for about 30 minutes to drain it; then put it in a in a baking tray
- Season the fish with spices and oil
- For the stuffing, use:
- 1/3 Cup of pine nuts or of shredded almonds
- 2 Tablespoons of olive oil
- 1 Cup of chopped parsley
- 3 Crushed garlic cloves
- 1 Pinch of allspice to taste

Directions:

1. Sauté the nuts into the oil until you obtain lightly brown nuts.
2. Add the parsley and the spices and sauté the ingredients for about 1 additional minute
3. Stuff the raw fish with the obtained mixture in order to prevent the fish from drying
4. Now, wrap the fish with a little bit of oil and bake it for about 30 minutes in the oven
5. Remove the fish from the oven; then serve and enjoy!

Nutritional information

- Calories per serving – 156.2 calories
- Fat per serving – 5.5 grams
- Saturated Fat – 1.2 grams
- Total Carbs per serving – 5.2 grams
- Protein per serving – 21.5 grams
- **NOTE:**

If you are eager to find more Vegetarian Recipes, we have a wide range of books that will enlighten you with various recipes. And in addition to the diversity of recipes; you will find all the information you need about a proper vegan diet.

CHAPTER 11

CONCLUSION

WE ARE REALLY happy to offer you this Paleo Diet book and we also hope that you will enjoy making the recipes that you will learn from this book. Please, if you enjoyed reading this material; feel free to share your ideas and if you have any helpful suggestions; feel free to share it with your friends. You are also able to help others find it in order to encourage us writing the books that you want to read.

www.ingramcontent.com/pod-product-compliance
Lightning Source LLC
Chambersburg PA
CBHW071214240726

48654CB00009B/775